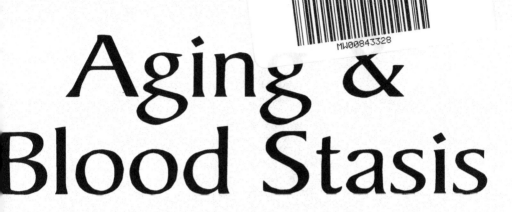

Aging & Blood Stasis

A New TCM Approach to Geriatrics

by Yan De-Xin

translated by
Tang Guo-shun
& Bob Flaws

BLUE POPPY PRESS
Portland, Oregon

Published by:

BLUE POPPY PRESS
A Division of Blue Poppy Enterprises, Inc.
4804 SE 69th Avenue
Portland, OR 97206

First Edition, June 1995
Second Printing, March, 2000
Third Printing, January, 2004
Fourth Printing, April, 2005
Fifth Printing, March, 2006
Sixth Printing, August, 2006
Seventh Printing, July, 2007
Eighth Printing, May, 2008
Nineth Printing, November, 2009
Tenth Printing, January, 2013
Eleventh Printing, January, 2014
Twelfth Printing, April, 2015
Thirteenth Printing, January, 2016
Fourteenth Printing, September, 2017
Fifteenth Printing, April, 2019
Sixteenth Printing, March, 2021

ISBN 0-936185-63-6
ISBN 978-0-936185-63-7
LC# 95-77296

DISCLAIMER: The information in this book is given in good faith. However, the author and the publishers cannot be held responsible for any error or omission. The publishers will not accept liabilities for any injuries or damages caused to the reader that may result from the reader's acting upon or using the content contained in this book. The publishers make this information available to English language readers for research and scholarly purposes only.

The publishers do not advocate nor endorse self-medication by laypersons. Chinese medicine is a professional medicine. Laypersons interested in availing themselves of the treatments described in this book should seek out a qualified professional practitioner of Chinese medicine.

COMP Designation: Functional translation using a standard translational terminology

22 21 20 19 18 17 16

Printed at Frederic Printing, Aurora, CO

Cover calligraphy by Michael Sullivan (Seiho)

Editor's Preface

This book is a functional translation of selected parts of Yan De-xin's *Zhong Guo Li Dai Zhong Yi Kang Shuai Lao Mi Yao (Secret Essentials for Combating Senility with TCM in China Through Various Dynasties)* published by the Literary Press in Shanghai in 1993. They have been translated by Dr. Tang Guo-shun and the current editor. Yan De-xin is one of the most famous *lao zhong yi* or old Chinese doctors in the People's Republic of China. A biography of his major accomplishments is found in the back of this book.

In particular, Prof. Yan is renowned for his special theory about the causation and treatment of senility. In Chinese, *shuai lao* (衰老) literally means the decline due to aging. Chinese-English medical dictionaries translate this as senility, but the reader should be cautioned that senility does not just mean mental senility but encompasses all the degenerative conditions, both physical and mental, associated with aging. As Prof. Yan points out, most Chinese medical texts down through the ages have emphasized that senility is due to vacuity of the spleen and/or kidneys. However, it is Prof. Yan's opinion and experience that senility is primarily due to static blood and the loss of balance between the qi and blood. In other words, it is Prof. Yan's theory that it is static blood which results in the vacuity detriment that is obvious in the elderly. Therefore, both his preventive regimes for promoting longevity and his remedial treatment of geriatric diseases are primarily based on rectifying the qi, quickening the blood, and transforming stasis. Prof. Yan calls this method of treatment, *heng fa* (衡法) or the balancing method.

We believe this book is a valuable addition to the English language literature on Traditional Chinese Medicine (TCM) for three reasons. First, it presents effective treatments for a variety of geriatric diseases based on the life-long experience of an old Chinese doctor who is renowned throughout China. Thus this book is a repository of clinically efficacious, empirically tested formulas. Secondly, this book is an example of the continual development of TCM. Although Prof. Yan cites the classics over and over again as he lays the groundwork for his theory and treatment of senility, nevertheless, the conclusions he comes to are new and revolutionary. This helps underscore the fact that TCM is not some dinosaur or relic from the past which has miraculously survived into the present but is a vital, continually growing, and alive system of thought and health care.

Third, this book is an excellent example of the TCM thought process. Prof. Yan comes to his conclusions and supports his theses by quoting a succession of basic statements of fact within TCM. It is this manipulation of such statements of fact that characterizes the logic of TCM. Because this logic is, to a great extent, dependent upon the Chinese language, it is my experience that Western practitioners of this methodology often have a hard time making it work. Hopefully this book will provide an example for Western practitioners of TCM of how Chinese practitioners think within this system so that we can model our own thought-processes within TCM upon that logic more closely. This is the thought process that has been honed and shown to work over 2,000 years by expert Chinese practitioners, and if we abandon this methodology or misapply it, we risk cutting ourselves off from that 2,000 years of experience. Western practitioners interested in developing a repertoire of basic TCM statements of fact should see my *Statements of Fact in Tradtional Chinese Medicine*, Blue Poppy Press, Boulder, CO, 1994.

Readers interested in a more standard approach to the TCM diagnosis and treatment of geriatric diseases are recommended to see Anna Lin's and my *The Dao of Protecting Health & Increasing Longevity* published by Blue Poppy Press, Inc., Boulder, CO, 1991. That book discusses what has been, up until recently the accepted TCM theory on aging, the

TCM principles of disease prevention and nourishing longevity for the elderly, and the diagnosis and treatment of the most common geriatric diseases based on TCM pattern discrimination. Because Dr. Yan combines his approach with TCM pattern discrimination, this current book and that one complement and augment each other.

This book has been translated using a standard Chinese medical terminology as it appears in Nigel Wiseman's *Glossary of Chinese Medical Terms and Acupuncture Points* published by Paradigm Publications, Brookline, MA, 1990. The major exception to this is that we have translated the word *luo* (络) as network vessels rather than connecting vessels based on a revised list of terms supplied to me by Dr. Wiseman. We have also translated several compound terms more literally than they usually are. For instance, *ying yang* (营 养) as a compound term means simply nutrition. However, when one understands that nutrition in the Chinese mind is made up from the words for construction and nourishment, I think this makes this concept within TCM all the more clear. Similarly, one might simply translate *xue liu yun xing* (血流运行) as the circulation of blood. However, if one translates it as the transportation and movement of blood, I believe this also elicits resonances which make this concept richer and more understandable from the TCM point of view.

The medicinal identifications in this book are based on Bensky & Gamble's *Chinese Herbal Medicine: Materia Medica* published by Eastland Press, Seattle, WA, 1986; Hong-yen Hsu's *Oriental Materia Medica: A Concise Guide* published by Oriental Healing Arts Institute, Long Beach, CA, 1986; *A Barefoot Doctor's Manual* published by Cloudburst Press, Seattle, WA, 1977; Stuart & Read's *Chinese Materia Medica* published by Southern Materials Center, Taipei, 1911; and the *Zhong Yao Da Ci Dian (Great Dictionary of Chinese Medicinals)* compiled by the Jiangsu New Medicine College and published by the Shanghai Science & Technology Press, Shanghai, 1991. In the few instances where all these resources have failed to enable us to make an identification of a medicinal given by Prof. Yan, we have identified those medicinals in Pinyin followed by the Chinese characters in parentheses. Prof. Yan gives specific instructions for the use of processed medicinals in certain formulas. Readers interested in learning about such processed medicinals and their clinical application should see Philippe Sionneau's *Pao Zhi: An Introduction to the Use of Processed Chinese Medicinals* published by Blue Poppy Press, Boulder, CO, 1995.

Identification of medicinal ingredients in formulas mentioned in this book but not included in the text is based on Dan Bensky & Randall Barolet's *Chinese Herbal Medicine: Formulas & Strategies*, Eastland Press, Seattle, WA, 1990; Margaret A. Naeser's *Outline Guide to Chinese Herbal Patent Medicines in Pill Form*, Boston Chinese Medicine, Boston, MA, 1990; and the *Jian Ming Zhong Yi Ci Dian (A Simple, Clear Chinese Medical Dictionary)* compiled by the Chinese National TCM Research Institute & the Guangzhou College of TCM and published by the People's Health & Hygiene Press, Beijing, 1986. Western medical terminology is based on the *Han Ying Chang Yong Yi Xue Ci Hui (A Chinese-English Collection of Commonly Used Medical Terms)* by Huang Xiao-kai *et al.*, published by the People's Health & Hygiene Press, Beijing, 1979.

This book is a functional translation because it is only a partial translation. The parts that appear are actually mostly denotative translations. However, because we have not identified exactly which parts are from which sections of Prof. Yan's original, Chinese language book, we can only call this a functional translation overall. Prof. Yan, through a Chinese-American intermediary, supplied Blue Poppy Press with a Chinese copy of his book *Zhong Guo Li Dai Zhong Yi Kang Shuai Lao Mi Yao* plus numerous pages of additional material in not very good English. Unfortunately, because we did not have a Chinese version of this added material to use in order to edit what was supplied to us and because the translation had major problems, after much soul-searching, we decided to include in this volume only material whose accuracy we could check ourselves from the Chinese.

In our opinion, most of what we have omitted is superfluous for the purposes of our perceived readership. The material omitted reiterates and expands the literary cites substantiating Prof. Yan's theories about static blood and discusses the history of Chinese thought on senility and geriatrics dynasty by dynasty. It is obvious that Prof. Yan would like to promote his new theory as widely in the world as possible and he argues his case at great length and often redundantly. It is clear from these arguments that he faces certain opposition in his own country. In addition, it appears that he hopes to reach practitioners of modern Western medicine as well as those of TCM. However, our readership has other needs and we feel that a complete rendering of Prof. Yan's book might be interesting to medical sociologists and anthropologists but not to the average Western practitioner of TCM.

That being said, in this book we have tried to present to Western practitioners of TCM is what we believe to be the clinically useful pith of Prof. Yan's theories and treatments. It is our belief that many of the arguments that Prof. Yan makes for his Chinese readership are unnecessary for our readership. We believe we have chosen a good and adequate presentation of Prof. Yan's case for emphasizing the role of static blood in aging and geriatrics. Ultimately, we believe that our readership is primarily interested in Prof. Yan's specific treatments for geriatric diseases. Therefore, the treatment section of Prof. Yan's original book forms the core of this book. In any case, I take personal responsibility for the choices of material that have been made in creating this book. May this book help promote and clarify the practice of TCM geriatrics in the Western world.

Bob Flaws
Feb. 24, 1995

Author's Preface

I have served as a physician for 54 years. During my middle age, I devoted myself to researching blood diseases. For a long time, I was absorbed in observing the blood. Through that observation, I discovered that the motion and quality of blood flow in the middle-aged is different from that in the elderly. Since then, through both literary research and clinical experience, I have come to the conclusion that static blood is the chief mechanism of senility. This conclusion has upset the traditional TCM theory handed down for several thousand years which holds that vacuity detriment is the chief cause of senility. This new theory has tremendously shaken TCM circles in China. Large numbers of clinical surveys, laboratory research, and animal experiments support this new point of view which is full of vitality and vigor.

This viewpoint has obtained proof and approval from Chinese medical pharmacologists, practitioners of integrated Chinese-Western medicine, and TCM practitioners at all levels. This new theory has also won the National Science & Technology in Chinese Medicinals Prize as well as the Prize for Excellence in Scientific & Technological Achievement at the National Medicine & Pharmacology Exhibition. In addition, the Shanghai Scientific & Educational Movie Works have produced a motion picture titled *Combating Senility: Qi, Blood & Longevity* based on this theory which has been shown around world in eight languages. Therefore, the influence of this theory has been wide.

Guided by this theory and based on the treatment principle in the *Nei Jing (Inner Classic)* that, "Peace is caused by dispersing qi and blood so as to regulate and transport them", I have selected various medicinals for the formulation of a number of prescriptions which have been used in clinical experiments. In this way, I and my associates have obtained large amounts of data. Based on this data, it is my belief and experience that, "Life destiny lies in transportation and stirring (*i.e.*, movement)" and "Life destiny lies in balance." In addition, I believe that further research confirming this approach to delaying senility is of utmost practical significance. Therefore, from 1992-3, I devoted myself to tracing the ancient literary sources of this theory, thus laying the groundwork for the systematic presentation of this approach to geriatrics and gerontology. Every step in this process has given me both great consolation that I am on the right track and great encouragement to continue my research into the role of static blood and aging.

To date, my students and I have written two books titled *Kang Shuai Lao—Qi Xue Yu Chang Shou (Combating Senility: Qi, Blood & Lengthening Longevity)* and *Zhong Guo Li Dai Zhong Yi Kang Shuai Lao Mi Yao (Secret Essentials in Combating Senility with TCM in China Through Various Dynasties)*. These books have been warmly welcomed by readers at home and abroad and have met with enthusiastic response. In addition, they have won the Prize for Progress in Science & Technology in the Municipal Health Department. During this time, I have also accepted invitations to lectures in Hong Kong, Taiwan, and the United States of America. Through reports in newspapers, magazines, and on radio and television, the fact that Chinese medicinals can make one healthy and long-lived has gone deep into the minds of the people all over the world. Thus I have received letters from different parts of the world asking me to compile a book on combating senility which is suitable for English-speaking readers. This book has, therefore, been specially prepared for publication in English. It is based on sections of my Chinese language book, *Zhong Guo Li Dai, Zhong Yi Kang Shuai Lao Mi Yao (Secret Essentials of Combating Senility with TCM in China Through Various Dynasties)*. I sincerely hope that all people under heaven may be blessed with longevity.

Yan De-xin
Dec. 1, 1993

Table of Contents

Editor's Preface v

Author's Preface xi

1 The Relationship of Qi and Blood to Senility 1

2 Master Yan's Diagnosis of the Pattern of Static
Blood 49

3 The Relationship Between the Symptoms of Senility
and Static Blood 59

4 Quickening the Blood & Regulating the Qi as an
Effective Method for Combating Senility 75

5 The Clinical Application of the Balancing Method . 79

6 Formulas for Combating Senility & Preserving Health
Based on the Balancing Method 93

7 Secret Essentials in the Treatment of Commonly
Seen Geriatric Patterns 105

8 Secret Essentials in the Treatment of Commonly
Seen Geriatric Diseases 175

9 Conclusion 247

Index 251

1
The Relationship of Qi & Blood to Senility

In Chinese, *yang sheng* means to nourish or prolong life and within Traditional Chinese Medicine (TCM) there is a large literature on the theories and methods of prolonging life. However, most of the theories and methods promulgated in the past for the prolongation of life and combating of senility are based on the theory of vacuity and repletion. This means that most previous TCM writers on geriatrics and gerontology have emphasized kidney vacuity, spleen vacuity, or spleen/kidney dual vacuity. Traditional senility-combating formulas almost all stress supplementation. Some supplement yin, others supplement yang, and yet others supplement both yin and yang. However, in their final analysis, they do not go beyond the scope of the theory on vacuity detriment in the viscera and bowels.

Based on my many years of clinical experience, I have come to the realization that vacuity detriment of the viscera and bowels does not fully describe the causes and conditions of human senility. Through research and observation, I have discovered that:

1) Human birth, growth, youthful vigor, and the decline and debility of aging are all related to the qi and blood.

2) The chief mechanism of senility is loss of regulation and harmony of the qi and blood.

3) This disharmony is mainly due to blood stasis.

As an extension of this realization, by applying the balancing method (*heng fa*), *i.e.*, the methods of quickening the blood and rectifying the qi, one may obtain marked effects in combating senility.

As the creator of this *heng fa* or balancing method, I have developed and refined this method through constant practice. Based on the viewpoint that, "Life consists of transportation and stirring (*i.e.*, movement)" and "Life consists of balance", I have come to the conclusion that "Phlegm and stasis have a common origin" and that "Boosting the qi transforms stasis." Based on these conclusions, I have selected Chinese medicinals to quicken the blood, open the network vessels, rectify the qi, and transform phlegm in the preparation of excellent formulas, such as *Heng Fa Chong Ji* (Balancing Method Soluble Preparation) and *Heng Fa Sheng Fang* (Balancing Method Sagelike Formula). Through clinical and experimental research, marked effects have been obtained using this method in preventing and eliminating stasis. Below is a description of the relationship of the theory of qi and blood to senility as well as the theoretical basis and clinical effects of this balancing method.

The Physiological Functions of Qi & Blood in the Human Body

Qi and blood are the basic substances which constitute the human body and maintain the activities of human life. Qi is the material basis for the normal physiological manifestations and life activities of the human body. Qi produces the functions of the different tissues and organs. Blood possesses the function of constructing and nourishing as well as enriching and moistening the whole body. It moves within the vessels, internally to the viscera and bowels, externally to the skin and flesh, sinews and bones. These circulate ceaselessly like an endless circle. Thus qi and blood maintain the normal physiological function of the human body. If a person has life, it is because of the person's normal physiological functions, and qi and blood play an essential role in those functions. Hence there are the ancient sayings, "What humans possess is but qi and blood" and "A human's blood, qi, essence, and spirit are what maintain their life."

Qi and blood are interdependent and closely interrelated. Physiologically, they promote each other in such a way that the viscera and bowels, sinews and bones, the four limbs, and the skin and hair all receive sufficient constructive nourishment and perform their functions. Pathophysiologically, qi and blood also affect each other. If the one is diseased, the other will be affected. Hence pathological changes occur leading to loss of regulation in the function of the viscera and bowels, frequent attack of various diseases, and eventually senility.

What qi means within TCM

Qi is an important concept in the history of Chinese philosophy. The theory of qi originates with the Daoists who thought that qi constitutes the most primitive substance among the tens of thousands of things between heaven and earth. This means that all the things in the universe result from changes in the motion of qi. It is this simple, materialistic viewpoint, combined with the experiences of ancient physicians and ideas from various other premodern Chinese sciences, such as astronomy/astrology, geomancy, and meteorology, that has formed the theory of qi as it is understood in TCM. This concept of qi had already been introduced to Chinese medicine as early as 2,000 years ago in the *Huang Di Nei Jing (The Yellow Emperor's Inner Classic)*. Today it forms one of the central concepts of TCM.

Traditional Chinese Medicine holds that the world is formed by qi and that humans also grow by receiving the qi between heaven and earth. The *Su Wen (Simple Questions)* says, "Humans depend for existence on the qi between heaven and earth and on the law of the four seasons." It also states:

> Humankind is born on earth, while our life depends on heaven. When the qi gathers between heaven and earth, humans comes into existence.

Qi is the material basis for maintaining the activities of human life. Qi in the body is a minute substance invisible to the naked eye. This minute substance possesses the characteristics of constant change and motion. Like irrigation by a mist or dew, qi passes through the body to perform the numerous physiological functions of steaming the skin, filling the body, and moistening the hair. Ancient people referred to this process of motion and change as *qi hua* or qi transformation. It is due to the constant, unceasing function of qi transformation in the body that such matters as qi, essence, blood, fluids, and humors in the organism are normally produced, transformed, utilized, and discharged so as to meet the needs for the activities of one's life.

The production of qi

In the human body, there are different kinds of qi. However, the source and production of these different types of qi is nothing other than the essence qi in the kidneys, the essence qi from water and grain, and the clear qi in nature (*i.e.*, fresh air).

The essence qi in the kidneys is that former heaven or prenatal essence qi which is received from one's father and mother. This is hidden and treasured in the kidneys. It is the primordial matter that forms the human body and is known as the former heaven or prenatal qi. After birth, one's physiological functions depend for their foundation on the essence qi in the kidneys.

The essence qi from water and grain is the constructive and nourishing substance in food and drink dispersed and transformed (*i.e.*, digested) by the spleen and stomach. This is circulated throughout the whole body, internally to the viscera and bowels and externally to the skin and hair, the four limbs, the hundreds of bones, and wherever it may reach. It maintains the physiological activities of the organism and meets the needs for growth and development. The essence qi from water and grain is the common material basis for various other kinds of qi in the human body. It is the chief source of constructive and nourishing substances after one's birth. "The Treatise on the Five Flavors" in the *Ling Shu (Spiritual Pivot)* says: "If one does not take grain, qi will lessen within one day and become debilitated in half a month." This stresses the importance of the essence qi from water and grain in the activities of human life.

The clear qi is also called heaven's qi. It is that new, fresh, empty qi which is inhaled from nature into the body by the lungs. "The Treatise on Yin & Yang Signs" in the *Su Wen (Simple Questions)* states:

> Heaven's qi passes to the lungs. In one's lifetime, respiration through the lungs does not stop for a single moment. The qi exhaled from the lung is turbid, while that inhaled from nature is clear. The clear qi breathed into the lungs and the essence qi from water and grain transformed and engendered in the spleen are generally known as the "latter heaven qi."

In the process of one's life activities, former heaven and latter heaven qi mutually transform and engender, forming an inseparable whole. Without the filling and nourishment of the latter heaven qi, the former heaven qi becomes consumed, is exhausted and vanishes; while without the former heaven qi, the latter heaven qi is unable to be transformed and engendered and is hence unable to exist.

Thus it may be seen that the production of qi depends first on the supply of essence qi in the kidneys, essence qi from water and grain, and the clear qi inhaled, and secondly, on the normal functioning of the lungs, spleen, and kidneys.

Forms of qi movement

As a minute substance, qi has a very strong vital force. It incessantly pushes and stimulates the different physiological activities in the human body. It moves and circulates ceaselessly throughout the whole body. TCM has summarized the different modes of qi movement and stirring into its four most basic forms, namely, upbearing, downbearing, exiting, and entering.

These four forms of qi movement are chiefly reflected in the qi transformation and movement of the viscera and bowels. This movement is the basic characteristic of motion in life. Therefore, the upbearing, downbearing, exiting, and entering of qi pass through the whole process of life and constitute the outward appearance of the life activities of the human body. Conversely, once this motion stops, life also ceases. "The Great Treatise on the Six Minute Substances" in the *Su Wen (Simple Questions)* repeatedly emphasizes:

> Upbearing, downbearing, exiting, and entering, there is no place these do not function. If there is such a place, there engenderment and transformation stop. There they are scattered and divided.

> Where transformation and engenderment cease, there is no entering or exiting. If there is no exiting or entering, there is no upbearing and downbearing...

> If there is no exiting or entering, there will be no birth, growth, strength, old age, or end. If there is no upbearing and downbearing, there will be no birth, growth, transformation, harvest, or storage...

> If exiting and entering are abolished, the spirit mechanism will be transformed and extinguished. If upbearing and downbearing cease, qi will be orphaned and endangered.

The upbearing, downbearing, exiting, or entering of the qi mechanism is reflected in the functional activities of the viscera and bowels. The manifestations of these four motions of the qi mechanism are mutually harmonized and coordinated in the various viscera and bowels. Upbearing and downbearing mutually become each other's cause and serve each other. The five viscera store the essence qi which should be upborne, while the six bowels conduct the transformed matter which should be downborne. However, even among the five viscera, the qi should not only upbear but also downbear.

For instance, the liver should upbear the qi on the left, while the lungs should downbear the qi on the right. Heart fire descends into kidney water. Kidney water ascends to heart fire. The spleen and stomach are in the middle, connecting the upper and lower parts. They are capable of upbearing the clear qi and downbearing the turbid qi. They serve as the pivot for the upbearing and downbearing of the qi mechanism. Although the six bowels are mainly responsible for circulation and should downbear the qi, yet there may also be upbearing within this downbearing, for instance, the small intestine's absorption and reception of the finest essence and its effect on fluids and humors. As far as a single viscus is concerned, the liver mainly rules upbearing and emission but, at the same time, it governs coursing and discharge. Thus it is a single unit which can both upbear and downbear.

In this way, the upbearing, downbearing, exiting, and entering of the qi mechanism of the viscera and bowels in humans are mutually linked, coordinated, and harmonized. Only thus can the qi enter, exit, upbear, and downbear incessantly. Hence the qi mechanism reaches in an orderly fashion, smoothly and without inhibition, and this maintains the uniformity of the internal and external environments in the organism. This also insures the metabolism of matter within the organism as well as the dynamic balance in the transformation of energy.

The physiological functions of qi

1. The function of qi transformation

This refers to the mutual transformation of essence, qi, blood, and fluids and humors as well as the functional activities of the viscera and bowels. For instance, the formation of qi, blood, fluids, and humors requires the transformation of food and drink into the essence qi from water and grain. This is then again transformed into qi, blood, fluids and humors. This activity is a concrete reflection of qi transformation which operates continuously throughout one's life from beginning to end. The activities of qi transformation are centered in the five viscera, while the six bowels serve as auxiliaries. These activities depend on the true qi for stimulation and their foundation is dependent upon *yuan* or original yin. Human metabolism and organic activity, including internally circulation, digestion, absorption, and secretion and externally, vision, hearing, talking, and motion, all result from qi transformation.

2. The function of propulsion

Human growth and development, the physiological activities of the various viscera and bowels, the circulation of blood, and the diffusion of fluids and humors all depend on qi for stimulation and propulsion. This propelling function of qi enables all the nutritional substances to diffuse throughout the whole body so as to maintain normal human physiological activity. If this propelling function of qi is reduced, growth and maturity will be retarded and the function of the internal organs will also be decreased.

3. The function of warming

"The 22nd Difficulty" in the *Nan Jing (Classic of Difficulties)* says, "Qi is responsible for warming." It is the source of heat in the human body. Under the influence of qi warming, different tissues and organs such as the channels and network vessels and the viscera and bowels can carry on their normal physiological activities. Liquid matter, such as blood and fluids, also rely on warming to carry on their normal circulation. "The Treatise on Original Spirit" in the *Ling Shu (Spiritual Pivot)* states:

Qi is kept to warm the muscles, strengthen the skin, and fatten the sweat pores. Thus it is responsible for opening and closing the tissues.

If the function of warming is not sufficient, this may lead to a decline in the function of various viscera and bowels in the human body.

4. The function of defense

Qi performs the function of guarding the muscles and exterior, defending them against external evils. "The Treatise on Original Spirit" in the *Ling Shu (Spiritual Pivot)* says, "If the defensive qi is harmonious, the divisions of the articulation of the muscles will be uninhibited, the skin will be warm and soft, and the interstices will be tight." Because the interstices of the skin are tight, external evils cannot easily invade the body. If the muscles are invaded by external evils and if the qi is able to struggle with such disease evils and drive them out, then the human body may be restored to health.

5. The function of securing & containing

Qi is able to control the blood and prevent its spillage externally from the blood vessels. In this sense, qi may be likened to a dike, while blood may be compared to water. If the dike is firm, water will not leak in. Similarly, if qi secures, blood cannot move recklessly. In addition and in the same way, qi is also able to secure and contain the sweat, urine, saliva, and semen as well as the liquid in the stomach and intestines. The functions of qi of securing and containing and those of pushing and propelling counteract, support, and coordinate with each other. These enable qi to regulate and control the normal circulation, secretion, and discharge of liquids within the body. If qi becomes vacuous, it may not only reduce the function of propulsion, thus retarding the circulation of blood and produce blood stasis, but it may also lead to a decline in the function of securing and containing the blood. Hence blood may spill from the blood vessels resulting in hemorrhaging.

6. The function of reproduction

Human growth, development, decline due to old age, and reproduction all mainly depend upon the function of kidney qi. The kidney qi is transformed from kidney essence and is also known as kidney yang. Kidney qi is the source of the material basis and functional activities of the human body. Only when one is full of kidney qi can human vitality grow vigorously and have the ability to proliferate offspring.

7. The function of balance

Balance means that it is qi which is responsible for maintaining the dynamic equilibrium within the human body and coordinating it to function as an organic whole. The human body is composed of various organs, and each internal organ has its own physiological functions. Qi circulates in the whole body. It upbears, downbears, and goes wherever it may reach. Thus viscera and bowels are mutually coordinated and restricted by qi, forming a whole system of physiological function in the human body and maintaining the dynamic equilibrium of coordination and unity in the human body.

As described above, within the human body, qi is responsible for seven types of functions. These not only coordinate with but also supplement each other. Thus metabolism is enabled to proceed normally, and a person is able to live a long, healthy life.

The five types of qi

Because qi is distributed in different parts of the body and the qi in these different parts have their own characteristics, therefore one can name different types of qi. For instance, qi concentrated in the upper burner or chest is called ancestral qi. That gathered in the middle burner is called the central qi. That concentrated in the lower burner and originating from the kidneys is known as the original qi. *Wei qi* or defensive qi is emitted from the interstices of the skin, while *ying qi* or constructive qi circulates within the blood vessels.

1. Original qi

This is also known as source qi, true qi, and life qi. Of the different kinds of qi in the human body, it is the most important and fundamental. Original qi is acquired prenatally and is hidden and treasured within the kidney essence. It passes through the three burners and spreads to the whole body. Internally, it spreads to the viscera and bowels, while externally it spreads to the interstices of the skin and muscles. It goes wherever it may reach. It both stimulates the functional activities of the viscera and bowels and enriches and nourishes the four limbs and the hundreds of bones. Therefore, if the original qi is sufficient, the functions of the viscera and bowels are vigorous and resistance to disease will be strong. One will be healthy and long-lived. Conversely, if original qi is insufficient, the functions of the viscera and bowels will decline and resistance to disease will be weakened. Diseases may occur one after another and may finally result in early death. Thus, we should pay attention to preserving our original qi while we are still healthy; while in treatment, one should stress the importance of cultivating and supplementing the original qi. This is very important in preventing and treating disease as well as in delaying senility.

2. Ancestral qi

This is also known as the great qi and as chest qi. The ancestral qi is composed of the clear qi inhaled into the lungs from nature and combined with the essence qi from water grain which is transported and transformed by the spleen and stomach. The ancestral qi accumulates in the chest from where it diffuses throughout the entire body. It has two great physiological functions. The first is circulation in the respiratory tract. In terms of this, ancestral qi is responsible for breathing. Language, sound, and the strength or weakness of breathing are all connected with the exuberance or decline of the ancestral qi. The second is the flow of qi and blood through the heart vessels. Thus the circulation of blood is also related to the ancestral qi. Through respiration and the circulation of blood, the ancestral qi is connected to the functional activities of the whole body. In his *Du Yi Sui Bi (Notes on the Study of Medicine)*, Zhou Xue-hai states:

> The ancestral qi is the stirring qi. Respiration, speech, sound, the motion of the limbs, and the strength or weakness of sinews and bones are all due to the operation of ancestral qi. If it is vacuous, the breath will be short and scant. If it is replete, there will be panting and wheezing, distention and fullness."

3. The central qi

The central qi is also known as the stomach qi. Its chief source is from food and drink. It is produced through the rottening and ripening of the stomach and is transported and transformed by the spleen. All the viscera and bowels in the human body require their supply of central qi in order to maintain their different physiological functions. "The Treatise on the *Tai Yin & Yang Ming*" in the *Su Wen (Simple Questions)* states:

> The four limbs receive their qi from the stomach. Sometimes, the spleen qi does not reach the channels due to disorder of the spleen. As a result, it cannot move the fluids and humors of the stomach. The four limbs thus do not obtain qi from water and gain. Hence the qi is gradually weakened. The circulation in the vessels is not smooth, and the sinews, bones, and muscles all lack the qi to exist; so they cannot function well.

In his "Treatise on the Exuberance & Decline of the Spleen & Stomach" in the *Pi Wei Lun (Treatise on the Spleen & Stomach)*, Li Dong-yuan also states:

> When food and drink enter the stomach, the yang qi goes upward. The fluids and humors and qi enter the heart, pass through the lungs, fill and make replete the skin and hair, and scatter in the hundreds of blood vessels. The spleen receives qi from the stomach and sprinkles to the four sides, nourishing qi and blood... Humans receive the qi of water and grain and live. This is rooted in their stomach qi.

Because the central qi rottens and ripens food and drink in order to obtain nutrition for the body, so it also enriches and constructs the defensive and constructive and the viscera and bowels. It upbears the clear and downbears the turbid, transports and transforms in the four directions. Hence, various masters of TCM in different generations have regarded the spleen and stomach as root of latter heaven.

4. The constructive qi

The constructive is made from the finest essence of the water and grain qi and it moves within the vessels. Thus it makes up a part of the circulation of blood. Its main function is the transformation and engenderment of the blood and body fluids and it follows the circulation of blood to construct and nourish the entire body. Because the constructive qi and blood move together within the vessels, day and night without pause they transport and move above and below, to the interior and exterior, to the viscera and bowels, and to the four limbs and the hundreds of bones in order to provide all these with nutrition. Therefore the constructive and the blood are often mentioned together.

5. The defensive qi

The defensive qi is a part of the yang qi in the human body. Therefore, it is also known as defensive yang. Its original source comes from the yang qi in the kidneys. However, it must depend on the latter heaven finest essence of water and food for constant nourishment. This essence is produced after birth in the spleen and stomach. Then the defensive qi is circulated through the body by the diffusion and emission of qi from the lungs. Therefore, it can be said that the defensive qi originates from the lower burner, is enriched and nourished in the central burner, and is opened and emitted from the upper burner. This qi is transported and moves outside the vessels and throughout the entire body. It performs the function of guarding and defending the muscles and exterior, defending these against external evils, opening and closing the sweat pores, regulating the body temperature, moistening the skin and hair, and warming the viscera and bowels.

In addition, each viscus and bowel has its own qi. For instance, the liver has its qi for growth and development. It is responsible for coursing and discharge. The heart has its qi of fire and warmth. It rules growth and nourishment. The spleen has its qi of water and grain. It governs transportation and transformation. The lungs have their qi to clear and depurate. It governs administration and discipline. The kidneys have their qi to store the essence of life. It governs the regulation of water metabolism and the control and promotion of respiration. It also determines the condition of the bones and marrow. Physiologically, each of these various types of visceral qi have their own functional characteristics. Thus, when one or another of the viscera become diseased, different symptoms appear.

The function of blood within TCM

Blood is an essential substantial matter for the formation of the human body. It performs the physiological functions of constructing and nourishing and enriching and moistening the tissues and organs of the entire body. Blood circulates ceaselessly in the vessels, internally to the five viscera and six bowels and externally to the skin and flesh, sinews and bones. It constantly moves without cessation throughout the entire body with its viscera and bowels and various tissues so as to fully fulfill its functions of constructing and nourishing and enriching and moistening and thus maintain normal physiological activities.

What blood means within TCM

Blood refers to the red liquid circulating within the vessels. The five viscera are formed during gestation when blood has already begun to circulate in the vessels of the whole body. This blood comes from the mother's body. After birth, the source of blood comes from food which is transformed and engendered by the function of qi transformation. The chief function of blood is to circulate in the vessels and construct and nourish the whole body. Thus, if a person has blood, there is life. If a persons loses blood, there will be disease. And if a person is without blood, there is death. Zhang Jie-bin, in his *Jing Yue Qian Shu (The Complete Writings of Jing-yue)* states:

> The intelligence of each of the seven portals, the movement of the four limbs, the harmony and softness of the sinews and bones, the abundance and exuberance of the muscles and flesh, the enrichment of the viscera and bowels, the calmness of the spirit, the moistness of the color of the cheeks, the filling of the constructive and defensive, the free flow and movement of the fluids and humors, the free flow and lack of inhibition of the two yin, none of these functions can occur without abundant blood. In short, wherever there is form or substance in the human body, all depend upon the blood. For instance, if blood declines, the form will wither. If blood is vanquished, the form is ruined. Whether the hundreds of bones are on the exterior or in the interior (*i.e.*, no matter where in the body), wherever the blood is deficient, there disease will be observed.

The production of blood

The spleen and stomach are the source of qi and blood engenderment and transformation. It is pointed out in the chapter titled "Determining the Qi" in the *Ling Shu (Spiritual Pivot)*:

> The central burner receives qi from the juice (*i.e.*, chyme). It is transformed, becomes red, and is called blood.

This underscores that the basic substance in blood is the finest essence of grain and water transformed and engendered in the spleen and stomach. The *Jing Yue Quan Shu (The Complete Writings of Jing-yue)* also points out:

> Blood is the essence qi of water and grain. It wells up continuously and comes, but, in fact, it is engendered and transformed by the spleen.

Thus, it is obvious that TCM had already realized the relation of nutritious substances to the production of blood and also the function of the spleen to this production.

Kidney essence and bone marrow may also be transformed into blood. "The Treatise on the Engendering of Qi Communicating with Heaven" in the *Su Wen (Simple Questions)* says, "If the bone marrow is hard and secure, qi and blood will follow it." In the *Bing Ji Sha Zhuang (Disease Mechanism Sand Seal)*, it is said, "The source of blood is in the kidneys." This clearly shows that the production of blood is related to the kidneys' treasuring of essence and that the kidneys rule the function of the engenderment of the bones and marrow. Essence and marrow are the raw materials for the engenderment and transformation of the blood, while the bones are the foundation for the blood's engenderment and transformation. If essence is sufficient, blood is also effulgent. If marrow is full, blood is not deficient. Hence the kidneys are an important organ in ensuring the production of blood.

The liver is responsible for storing and engendering the blood. "The Treatise on the Appearances of the Six Bowels" of the *Su Wen (Simple Questions)* says, "The liver...filled with sinews, engenders qi and blood." This clearly explains that the liver is not only an organ for storing the blood but is also capable of engendering the blood. In the process of producing blood, the liver further requires the mutual coordination and close cooperation of the other organs. The *Zhang Shi Yi Tong (Master Zhang's Medical Knowledge)* states:

> If qi is not consumed, essence will be returned or gather in the kidneys and be made into essence. If essence is not discharged, it will gather in the liver and be transformed into clear blood.

This clearly shows how the liver and kidneys cooperate to transform essence in order to engender blood.

The heart and lungs also play an important role in the production of blood. "The Great Treatise on Yin & Yang Resonances & Appearances" in the *Su Wen (Simple Questions)* says, "The heart engenders blood." This points out that the heart has the functions of regulating, disciplining, harmonizing, and controlling the production of the blood. Once the heart viscus suffers damage, the spirit brilliance loses its uniform regulation, discipline, and control, thus affecting the production of blood. "The Treatise on the Engenderment & Reunion of the Constructive & Defensive" in the *Ling Shu (Spiritual Pivot)* states:

> The central burner is also in the stomach. After it exits from the upper burner, the qi received discharges the dross, steams the fluids and humors, transforms the finest essence, flows upward into the vessels of the lungs, and then transforms itself into blood.

Thus we may see that after water and grain are received and digested in the stomach, they are engendered and transformed into finest essence. Then this is transported through the spleen, is acted upon by qi transformation, steamed, upborne and downborne within the lungs so that the finest essence combined with fluids and humors becomes blood.

Characteristics of blood circulation

Blood circulates within the vessels. Pushed and stirred by the qi, it flows along the blood vessels to various parts of the entire body. It circulates or travels ceaselessly like an endless circle. This circulation of blood provides the various viscera and bowels and tissues of the entire body with rich nutritious substances so as to meet their needs in their performance of their functions.

Blood flows along in a relatively closed tube known as a *mai* or vessel. The thin or tiny vessels are called network vessels. These vessels and network vessels prevent the blood from flowing and spilling outside of the channels and thus causing various forms of hemorrhage. Throughout the activities of life, blood flows in a cyclic, uninterrupted manner. It circulates rhythmically along a definite route. "The Treatise on the Images of Qi of the Average Person" in the *Su Wen (Simple Questions)* says:

> When a person breathes in, the vessels surge or throb. When they breathe out, they throb again. When they inhale and exhale regularly, the pulse throbs 5 times. There is an interval for respiration. This is the condition of the average person.

Because the flow of blood has a certain rhythm, we may rely on the rhythm of breathing to make some calculations. If the pulse throbs more or less than 5 times (per respiration), this indicates a pathological state. "The Treatise on Distinguishing the Channels & Vessels" in the *Su Wen (Simple Questions)* states:

Food qi enters the stomach. The turbid qi gathers in the heart. The abundant essence enters the vessels. The vessel qi flows to the channels. The channel qi gathers in the vessels. The lungs face the hundreds of vessels. They transport the channels to the skin and hair. The hair and vessels combine with the essence and move the qi to the bowels. If the bowels' essence spirit is bright, it will be retained in the four treasuries. If qi gathers and is balanced, balance results in evenness. Thus the qi mouth at the *inch* (position) determines life and death.

Although the exact route of blood circulation described by the ancients is different from that in modern anatomy, it clearly points out that the heart, lungs, and vessels (with their pulse) constitute the blood circulatory system and marks out the route of travel from the heart, through the vessels to the lungs.

Thus the normal circulation of blood occurs through the mutual coordination of the heart, lungs, liver, and spleen. The heart governs the blood vessels. Heart qi is the basic, motive power which pushes the circulation of blood. It is mainly because of this action of pushing that blood circulates in the vessels in a definite direction. The lungs are in charge of respiration and govern the qi of the entire body. The lungs are indispensable for the production of ancestral qi, while the chief function of ancestral qi is to circulate blood and qi through the vessels of the heart. Hence it is clear that the normal circulation of blood has a close relationship with the lungs. The liver is responsible for storing the blood. This function of storing blood harmonizes, regulates, and disciplines the amount of blood in circulation. The liver also most definitely functions to keep the blood flow free-flowing and uninhibited. The spleen restrains the blood. It is able to restrain, contain and control blood so that it may not spill and exit outside the vessels.

Therefore, the normal flow of blood requires, first, a perfect system of healthy and tight vessels, and secondly, the propulsion and stirring of the relevant visceral qi. If the vessels and network vessels lose their security and tightness or the visceral qi is diseased, then the blood cannot move normally or transport and move uninhibitedly but rather there will be obstruction and stagnation within the vessels and depression internally within the body. This is known as blood stasis. It is also possible for flow exiting from the vessels and network vessels and even exiting and discharge to the outside of the body. This is called hemorrhage. Whether it is blood stasis or hemorrhage, all this is considered as "outside the channels blood." Since this blood has already left the vessels and network vessels, it loses the normal physiological function of the blood and becomes a pathological product.

The physiological functions of the blood

1. Moistening the four limbs & hundreds of bones, filling & nourishing the five viscera & six bowels

Blood is one of the most important substances for the construction and nourishing of the organism. A person's skin and hair, sinews and bones, and viscera and bowels all must obtain sufficient nourishment from the incessant circulation of blood. This then results in normal physiological function. For instance, when the eyes obtain blood, they can see. When the feet obtain blood, they can walk. When the palms obtain blood, they can grasp. When the sinews obtain blood, they do not wither. When the skin and hair obtain blood, they show pleasing colors. If the blood circulates ceaselessly, it sends the finest essence of nutrition throughout the entire body and enables the discharge of turbid waste matter from it. Therefore, blood is an essential requirement for the maintenance of the life of the organism.

2. Nourishing & fostering the heart spirit

Blood is the chief material basis of a human being's essence spirit (*i.e.*, mental/emotional) activities. The heart controls the blood. It also governs the spirit and orientation. When the heart is nourished by blood, the spirit becomes clear and orientation becomes acute. "The Treatise on the Eight Righteous Spirit Brilliances" in the *Su Wen (Simple Questions)* states:

> Blood and qi are a human's spirit. It is not all right to not be careful in nourishing them.

If one's essence spirit is full and abundant, the spirit orientation becomes clear and sober. One's sensations will be quick and nimble and one can move as one likes. All this depends upon the fullness and exuberance of the blood and the regular, harmonious, coursing and disinhibition of the blood vessels. If the blood loses its normalcy, then, in mild cases, there will be heart palpitations and forgetfulness and the essence spirit will wither. In severe cases, there will be senility or decline due to aging.

3. Maintaining the balance of yin & yang in the organism

Blood pertains to yin and qi pertains to yang. Disease changes in the blood may lead to the imbalance of yin and yang in the organism. In the *Xue Zheng Lun (Treatise on Bleeding Patterns)* it is said:

> In the human body, there is nothing outside of yin and yang, and these two words, yin and yang, mean water and fire. (While) the two words, water and fire, mean qi and blood.

Thus it may be seen that blood is an essential substance for maintaining the balance of yin and yang in the organism.

4. The reproductive function

When a woman grows to maturity, the *ren mai* is open and free-flowing, the *tai chong mai* is exuberant, the sea of blood is full, and menstruation descends periodically. After menstruation, the sea of blood is empty and vacuous. Therefore, the sea of blood again begins to store the blood. Eventually it becomes full again and afterwards the menstruation descends another time. Thus it repeats cyclically as long as the woman's normal physiological functions are maintained. Therefore, when blood becomes effulgent and exuberant, the menstruation is capable of periodically descending and the woman is capable of conceiving and giving birth. Conversely, if the blood is insufficient, the sea of blood will not be able to become periodically full and hence the woman will not be able to give birth.

The *Nan Jing (Classic of Difficulties)* describes the blood's constructing, nourishing, enriching, and moistening in a general way when it says, "The blood governs moistening." This clearly demonstrates that blood has a very important role in the maintenance of the activities of human life.

Interrelationships between the qi & blood

Qi and blood constitute the two great basic substances in maintaining the activities of the human body. Physiologically, these two substances are interrelated and inseparable. Pathologically, they also affect each other. They serve as cause and effect for each other. Therefore, TCM practitioners in ancient times said, "Blood and qi, different names, same category." Qi without blood is not harmonious, while blood without qi cannot move. The relationship between qi and blood may be summarized thus: "Qi is the commander of the blood" and "Blood is the mother of qi."

1. The effects of qi on the blood

Qi produces three effects on the blood. Namely, qi can engender the blood, qi can move the blood, and qi can contain the blood.

A. Qi is capable of engendering the blood

Qi is the motivating force in the production of blood. After the intake of food and drink, these are transformed into the finest essence of water and grain. Then they are turned into fluids and humors and constructive qi, and finally these are transformed into the red color of blood.

In this process of transformation, not a single step can be accomplished without the moving and transforming functions of qi. The *Du Yi Sui Bi (Notes on the Study of Medicine)* states:

> The human body has a kind of qi whose character and function can activate the blood in the human body. From a little bit to an enormous amount, where qi stops, blood also ceases to circulate. It is often seen that if a person's qi is scant or if their qi is damaged by diseases, then the colors of their face and network vessels will become pale, but they do not have any pattern of loss of blood. This is because their qi and strength have already become weak and are not capable of quickening and transforming the blood.

When qi is effulgent, the function of transforming and engendering the blood is strong. If qi is weak, then the ability and power to transform and engender the blood will also be diminished. In the clinical treatment of blood vacuity disease, it is common, therefore, to also use qi-supplementing medicinals so that the qi is able to engender the blood.

B. Qi is capable of moving the blood

Blood pertains to yin which is governed by quiet. It is not capable of moving itself. Therefore, it depends on the propulsion of qi. On the one hand, qi can directly propel the motion of the blood. On the other hand, by promoting the functional activities of the viscera and bowels, the blood is also cyclically coursed and moved. "The Treatise on the Production of the Five Viscera" in the *Su Wen (Simple Questions)* says, "Qi moves and then the blood flows." In the *Xue Zheng Lun (Treatise on Bleeding Patterns)* it is said, "That which circulates the blood is the qi." Thus it may be seen that the normal functioning of the qi plays a very important role in insuring the smooth circulation of blood.

C. Qi is capable of containing the blood

Qi is capable of securing and containing the flow of blood so that it moves within the channels and network vessels. Thus blood may circulate in the vessels uninterruptedly so as to supply substances for construction and nourishment to the various viscera and bowels and tissues of the entire body. If qi becomes diseased, it may not be able to contain the blood. In that case, the symptoms of hemorrhage will appear. Clinically, if there is the crisis of blood desertion, then root treatment consists of the great principle, "In case of blood desertion, secure the qi."

2. The effects of blood on the qi

A. Blood is capable of engendering the qi

Blood transports and moves ceaselessly, thus providing the finest essence of water and grain for the production and functional activities of qi. This finest essence of water and grain is the main material basis for the production of all the various kinds of qi in the entire body. Therefore the ancient saying goes, "Blood is the mother of qi." This means that the production of qi is always inseparable from blood. Thus the normalcy of the blood flow has a close relationship with the production of qi.

B. Blood is capable of carrying the qi

Blood is the carrier of the qi and qi is the transporter of blood to the entire body. If qi does not reside within the blood, it will float about unstably without any destination. Thus it is said, "Blood is the dwelling place of the qi." Clinically, in the aftermath of any appearance of great exiting of blood, qi will also follow and be scattered in its wake. Thus there emerges qi following blood desertion symptoms.

In short, qi is the commander of the blood, while blood is the mother of qi. Qi and blood, one is yin and one is yang and both are interrelated. Qi is blood without form, while blood is the form of qi. Qi includes within it the blood. The blood includes within it the qi. Therefore qi and blood are interdependent and circulate together uninterruptedly. If blood and qi are not harmonious, then hundreds of diseases may occur.

The Relationship of Qi & Blood to Combating Senility

Human physiology and pathophysiology, longevity and senility are all closely related to the qi and blood. With advancing years, qi and blood undergo pathological changes such as loss of balance and stasis and obstruction which may lead to the occurrence of various diseases and the senility of the organism. Therefore, in order to enjoy a healthy, long life, one must attach importance to the regulation and harmony of the qi and blood.

The relationship of qi & blood to physiological activities

Qi and blood are the most precious substances in the human body which is filled with these substances. Human physiological functions and physiological changes are normal because qi and blood are harmonious and the constructive and defensive are free-flowing. The chapter titled "Heaven's Decreed Years" in the *Ling Shu (Spiritual Pivot)* states:

> Blood and qi are harmonious. Constructive and defensive are free-flowing. The five viscera are produced. The spirit qi exists in the heart. The ethereal soul and the corporeal soul are formed. Thus do humans come into existence.

1. The relationship of qi & blood to essence, qi & spirit

Essence, qi, and spirit are the *san bao* or three treasures in the human body. They are the material basis for the normal physiological activities of the human body. The exuberance and decline of the essence, qi, and spirit are closely related to the qi and blood. No matter whether essence is prenatal or postnatal, its formation depends upon fullness and exuberance of the qi in the human body. If qi is exuberant, essence will also be full. If qi is weak, then essence will decline. Moreover, the physiological functions of essence also rely on qi for their propulsion and stimulation, while the secretion and treasuring of essence rely on the qi's securing and guarding. The *Lei Jing (Systematized Classic)* states:

> Essence and blood in the human body are transformed due to qi. Therefore qi gathers in the essence.

Blood is also capable of engendering essence. Blood flows into the kidneys. Within the kidneys it undergoes transformation and is stored in the kidneys as essence. Therefore, if blood is effulgent, essence is full. If blood is deficient, essence will be scanty. The *Zhu Bing Yuan Hou Lun (Treatise on the Origins & Symptoms of Various Diseases)* says, "The kidneys treasure, and essence is produced from the blood." The spirit is the outward manifestation of life activities in turn based on the qi and blood. The spirit can exist only on the basis of full and sufficient qi and blood. The spirit is embodied in the qi which is transformed into the spirit. If qi is exuberant, the spirit is effulgent. If qi declines, the spirit becomes scanty. If qi is severed, the spirit dies. The *Pi Wei Lun (Treatise on the Spleen & Stomach)* says, "Qi is the grandfather of spirit." Blood is the chief material basis for the activities of the spirit and orientation. Blood circulates in the vessels and enriches and nourishes the five viscera and six bowels, the four limbs, the hundreds of bones, and the nine portals. It brings about the activities of the spirit and ensures the normal physiological activities going on in various viscera and bowels and tissues of the entire body. Hence, if blood is exuberant, the spirit is effulgent. If blood is scant, the spirit becomes cowardly or nervous. If blood is finished, the spirit dies.

2. The relationship of qi & blood to the functional activities of the viscera & bowels

The normal functional activities of the viscera and bowels also depend on the functioning of the qi and blood. Qi has the function of warming and stimulating the various viscera and bowels. The chapter titled "Measuring the Vessels" in the *Ling Shu (Spiritual Pivot)* states:

> Without qi there is no movement. Like the flow of water and the ceaseless motion of the sun and moon, the yin vessels construct the viscera and the yang vessels construct the bowels. This repeats uninterruptedly from beginning to end like an endless circle. The flowing qi moistens internally the viscera and bowels and externally the interstices.

This shows that qi is not only the motivating force in the circulating blood but is also the substance for maintaining the functional activities of the viscera and bowels within the human body. Qi circulates internally and externally through every part of the body. It repeats this circulation from beginning to end just like a circle and provides the motivating force for the activities of the viscera and bowels and the various tissues within the human body. Thus it preserves the health of the human body.

Blood possesses the function of enriching and moistening the tissues of the viscera and bowels. The chapter titled "Root Treasuries" in the *Ling Shu (Spiritual Pivot)* says, "If blood is harmonious, then it courses and moves in the channels and vessels, constructing and restoring yin and yang, strengthening the sinews and bones, and clearing and disinhibiting the joints." This shows that blood is also the nutritional substance for the physiological activities of the tissues and the viscera and bowels.

Qi and blood warm, moisten, and nourish the viscera and bowels and channels and vessels and thus bring into full play their respective functions. "Measuring the Vessels" in the *Ling Shu (Spiritual Pivot)* states:

> The lung qi opens into the nose. If the lungs are harmonious, the nose is capable of knowing fetor and fragrance. The heart qi opens into the tongue. If the heart is harmonious, the tongue is capable of knowing the five flavors. The liver qi opens into the eyes. If the liver is harmonious, the eyes are capable of knowing and distinguishing the five colors. The spleen qi opens into the mouth. If the spleen is harmonious, the mouth is capable of knowing the five grains. The kidney qi opens into the ears. If the kidneys are harmonious, the ears are capable of hearing the five sounds.

The "Chapter on the Production of the Five Viscera" in the *Su Wen (Simple Questions)* states:

> The eyes receive blood and are capable of seeing. The feet receive blood and are capable of walking. The palms receive blood and are capable of grasping. The fingers receive blood and are capable of holding.

Thus we may think that qi and blood are the basic substances for maintaining the activities of human life and that they are the root of life in the human body.

The Balance of Qi & Blood and Its Relationship to Combating Senility

As has been said above, qi and blood are the two great basic substances constituting the human body and maintaining the activities in our life. If qi and blood work normally, then the viscera and bowels, sinews and bones, the four limbs, and the skin and hair can all obtain sufficient nutrition. In that case, the human body will be healthy and long-lived. In the chapter on "Longevity & Early Death, Strength & Weakness" in the *Ling Shu (Spiritual Pivot)* it says:

If blood and qi triumph in the body, longevity results. If they do not triumph, there will be early death."

The *Jing Yue Quan Shu (The Complete Writings of Jing-yue)* states:

Humans have yin and yang, namely, qi and blood. Yang governs qi. Therefore, if qi is complete, the spirit is effulgent. Yin governs blood. Hence, if the blood is exuberant, the body will be strong. These are just the things on which one's life depends.

Conversely, the chapter "Heaven's Decreed Years" in the *Ling Shu (Spiritual Pivot)* states:

If blood and qi are vacuous, the vessels will not be free-flowing. Thus true and evil will mutually attack each other. There will be chaos and this will lead to one's longevity being cut short in middle age.

This discussion points out that the normal function of the qi and blood has a close relationship with one's longevity and health. If the flow of the qi and blood is uninhibited and balanced, then the qi and blood form the basis of the body's normal physiological functions. This is because all the different kinds of physiological activities in the human body take qi and blood as their material basis. Thus if the qi and blood flow uninhibitedly, openly, and without obstruction and are dynamically balanced, then the normal transportation and movement due to the functioning of the viscera and bowels will be uninhibited, the metabolic processes of the organism will be uninhibited, and the engenderment and transformation of qi and blood will have no limit. Hence it is said in the "Treatise on Regulating the Channels" of the *Su Wen (Simple Questions)*, "If blood and qi are not mixed, the five viscera are quiet and stable" and "If blood and qi are mixed, diseases will simultaneously be produced in the body."

The normal coursing and free flow of the qi and blood in the body not only supply the constructing and nourishing substances to the organism but also carry out the function of linking the tissues to the viscera and bowels and coordinating the relationship between the kidneys and the viscera. Both human physiological functions and pathological changes are mainly centered in the five viscera, while the six bowels are their auxiliaries. These five viscera and six bowels are connected by the vessels and network vessels to the five senses, the nine portals, the four limbs, and the hundreds of bones. Thus the inside and the outside are connected as an organic, integrated whole. Therefore, if the qi and blood flow uninhibitedly, the viscera and bowels are harmonious and regulated and there is good health and long life. But if the qi and blood lose their regularity, then the viscera and bowels lose their harmony. Static blood and phlegm turbidity are engendered internally. This then leads to disease and eventually to the decline of aging and premature death.

The transportation and stirring of the qi is known as the qi mechanism. The activities which occur within a person's tissues and viscera and bowels and those which take place between these tissues all occur due to a unity of opposites where the activities of upbearing, downbearing, entering, and exiting jointly bring to completion the metabolic processes of the entire organism. These activities ceaselessly take in food from outside, and, through the functioning of qi transformation, upbear the clear essence, downbear the turbid, and absorb the finest essence to nourish the whole body. At the same time, these activities discard metabolic waste products outside the body so as to maintain the dynamic balance between the metabolism of matter and its conversion into energy. "A Different Treatise on the Channels & Vessels" in the *Su Wen (Simple Questions)* states:

> Drink enters the stomach. The essence qi flows out and is transported above to the spleen. The spleen qi scatters this essence which gathers above in the lungs. It flows through and is regulated by the water passageways and is transported below to the bladder. The water essence spreads to the four directions, while the five channels travel together.

The *Su Wen (Simple Questions)* also states:

> When food qi enters the stomach, its essence is scattered to the liver,
> and the sinews are filled with this qi. When food qi enters the stomach,
> turbid qi gathers in the heart, and essence fills the vessels. The vessel
> qi flows into the channels and this vessel qi gathers in the lungs. The
> lungs face the hundreds of vessels and transport essence to the skin
> and hair. The hair and vessels combine with the essence and move this
> qi to the bowels. If bowels have essence, the spirit is bright and is
> retained in the four viscera. Thus qi returns to balance.

This clearly points out that the dynamic balance of upbearing and
downbearing, transportation and movement of the qi mechanism of the
viscera and bowels is the key for maintaining normal physiological
function.

In order for blood to supply the construction and nourishment of the
tissues of the five viscera and six bowels, the five senses, nine portals,
four limbs, and hundreds of bones of the entire body normally, it must
flow uninterruptedly like an endless circle. This normal circulation of
blood should have two forces, namely the stirring or propelling force
and the containing and securing force. The propelling force is the
motivating power for blood circulation. It is embodied in the functions
of coursing and discharge of the heart, lungs, and liver. The containing
and securing force keeps the blood from spilling outside. This is
dependent on the spleen's containment of the blood and the liver's
storage of the blood. It is the coordination and balance of these two
forces that maintains the normal circulation of blood. If the propelling
force is insufficient, there may appear such changes as slow motion,
stagnation and choppiness, blood stasis, etc. If the containing and
securing force is insufficient, this may lead to the blood spilling outside
and the exiting of blood. This will lead to loss of normalcy of the
viscera and bowel function and the loss of health of the organism.

As regards the criteria of the state of health and the basic condition of the physiological activities of the normal organism, the ancients usually employed the term *zheng ping*, normal and average or *ping*, average, as general descriptions. For instance, "The Treatise on the Signs of an Average Person's Qi" in the *Su Wen (Simple Questions)* says, "The average person is not diseased." This refers to healthy people as average or literally level people. "The Treatise on Regulating the Channels" in the *Su Wen (Simple Questions)* also states:

> When yin and yang are level (*ping*), the body is full. If this remains unchanged at all times, then we may call the person an average (*i.e.*, healthy) person.

Here the term average or ordinary means balance. If the qi and blood are balanced, then its expression will be that person's physiological functions are normal. As "The Great Treatise on the Supreme Truth" in the *Su Wen (Simple Questions)* says, "When qi and blood are normal and balanced, long will be one's heavenly (decreed) destiny." The transportation and movement of blood depend on the command of the qi, while the quiet and warmth of the qi rely on the moistening of the blood. These two conditions are both antagonistic and mutually interdependent. Therefore, maintaining the relative balance between the qi and blood is the basic requirement for the health and longevity of the human body.

The fundamental principle of nourishing life and combating old age in Traditional Chinese Medicine is, "To level (or calm) yin and secrete (or hide) yang." Yin and yang form a dichotomy within the human body. The law governing the formation, growth, and development of the human body cannot be separated from yin and yang. Therefore, "The Treatise of the Engendering Qi Communicating with Heaven" in the *Su Wen (Simple Questions)* says, "The root of life (or engenderment) is yin and yang." "The Treatise on the Whole Form of Precious Life" of the *Su Wen (Simple Questions)* further says, "Humans have their form which cannot be separated from yin and yang." Under normal physiological conditions within the human body, these two poles, yin and yang, must maintain a dynamic balance. If one side inclines toward debility and the other towards fullness, then the normal physiological functions of the human body will become chaotic and a disease state will occur. "The Treatise on the Engendering Qi Communicating with Heaven" in the *Su Wen (Simple Questions)* clearly points out:

> When yin is level and yang is secreted, the essence spirit is then in order. When yin and yang are separated, essence spirit is terminated.

Thus it may be seen that the preservation of yin and yang in the human body in dynamic balance is an essential principle for nourishing life and maintaining its constant engenderment and transformation.

Blood Stasis, the Chief Cause of Senility

Qi and blood should move uninhibitedly within the body, flowing freely and not stagnating. If the transportation and movement of the qi and blood become slow and relaxed or obstructed and stagnant, this will lead to blood stasis within the body. This static blood will separate and not combine with the blood that constructs and nourishes the entire body. Not only will it fail to engender and transform fresh blood but it will also cause the qi and blood to lose their balance. In this case, signs of trouble in one's physiological function will appear. Physiological function will eventually become diminished and weakened. Blood stasis will necessarily be engendered. Pathological metabolic products, such as phlegm turbidity, and various other disease changes will follow in its wake and will finally lead to senility.

Imbalance of qi & blood as the cause of a variety of diseases

Qi and blood constitute the basic substances of the human body. They are the material basis for the physiological activities of the tissues, viscera and bowels, channels and network vessels, etc. Once qi and blood lose their normalcy, various pathological changes will occur in the human body.

Loss of harmony of the qi & blood as the main cause of disease

From the point of view of TCM theory, within the human body, the progression from birth, growth, development, and youthful vigor to senility is nothing but the process of change from strength to weakness and from exuberance to decline of the qi and blood. Although there are many forms of change from birth through growth, youth, old age and disease to death, yet, in the final analysis, these are all inseparable from changes in qi and blood. If qi and blood lose their harmony and the vessels and network vessels become static and obstructed, then phlegm turbidity will be engendered internally and may lead to a chain of pathological changes, such as heat, cold, vacuity, and repletion in the viscera and bowels.

For instance, if qi and blood in the heart lose their harmony, there may appear heart palpitations and shortness of breath aggravated by movement. The heart spirit will not be quiet and there will be insomnia, poor memory, and excessive dreams. If qi and blood in the lungs lose their harmony, there may occur cough and panting with copious phlegm which are also made worse by movement as well as spontaneous sweating, etc. If qi and blood in the spleen lose their harmony, the complexion will become sallow yellow. The four limbs will become weak and fatigued, and there will be abdominal distention after eating. The stools will be loose and there may be uterine bleeding or bloody stools. If qi and blood in the liver lose their harmony, there may appear fatigue, emotional depression, timidity, and both eyes may become dry. There may also be diminished vision, numbness in the extremities, lusterless nails, and spasms of the sinews and vessels. If qi and blood in the kidneys lose their harmony, there may appear low back soreness, weak knees, tinnitus, deafness, poor memory, worry and anxiety.

Moreover, diseases in the viscera and bowels can be passed through the channels and network vessels and vice versa. The one may become the cause or the effect of the other. When one viscus has a disease, it may spread to the other viscera and bowels, eventually leading to disease in a number of viscera and bowels. As it is said in "The Treatise on Regulating the Channels" in the *Su Wen (Simple Questions)*:

> The pathways of the five viscera all exit from the channels within which move the blood and qi. When qi and blood are not harmonious, the hundreds of diseases are transformed and engendered. Thus it is necessary to guard the channels.

It is further stated:

> If qi and blood become mixed up, yin and yang fight with each other. Qi becomes chaotic in the defensive, while blood counterflows in the channels. When blood and qi are separated, one becomes replete, while the other becomes vacuous. If blood mixes with yin and qi mixes with yang, then fright and mania will occur. If blood mixes with yang and qi mingles with yin, this causes the sacred mean...

> If blood and qi become mixed up, this produces repletion. If both blood and qi flow upward, there will be great inversion (*i.e.*, syncope).

Therefore, we may say that loss of harmony of the qi and blood manifests pathologically as disease within the human body and loss of regulation of viscera and bowels. These both have a close relationship with the production of various pathologic metabolic products, such as blood stasis and phlegm turbidity. They may also be linked with any pathological changes in the viscera and bowels. Thus, based on qi and blood pattern discrimination, one can understand the disease mechanisms of diseases in the human body. And, by coursing, freeing the flow, regulating, and harmonizing the qi and blood, one can regulate the functions of the viscera and bowels and the body's tissues, disperse and eliminate static blood, phlegm turbidity, and other such evils, and hence convert the pathological state into the normal physiological condition. Thus one can treat a variety of diseases and restore health of the organism. Grasping the key link of qi and blood should be considered as getting to the root.

Types of pathological loss of balance of the qi & blood

Physiologically, qi and blood are mutually linked. Pathologically, they also affect each other. This is manifested first in the fact that their disease causes are the same. External evils and the six environmental excesses, internal damage due to the seven emotions, and food and drink, phlegm, and static blood may all cause disease changes in the qi and the blood. In addition, in the course of diseases of the qi and blood, diseases of the qi will eventually affect the blood and diseases of the blood will eventually affect the qi. When qi and blood are affected by the same disease, they may be affected sequentially. In other words, sometimes qi disease comes first, while other times blood disease comes first. However, in the course of disease, these two are never isolated but always affect each other. As it is said in the *Shen Zhai Yi Su (Bequeathed Writings on Cautions & Abstentions)*, "Qi disease damages the blood, while blood disease damages the qi." Further, pathological changes in the qi and blood always manifest in loss of normalcy in the functions of the viscera and bowels.

When the qi and blood lose their balance, this commonly results in the pathological patterns of qi and blood vacuity weakness, qi vacuity and blood stasis, qi stagnation and blood stasis, qi counterflow and blood counterflow, joining and binding of phlegm and stasis, qi not containing the blood, and blood desertion and qi desertion.

1. Qi & blood vacuity weakness

Qi vacuity refers to decline and diminishment in the function of the viscera and bowels and to the lowering of resistance to disease. Because the production and spread of qi are closely related to the lungs, spleen, and kidneys, qi vacuity is commonly observed in these three viscera. Blood vacuity means insufficiency of constructing and nourishing blood in the body. The engenderment and transformation of blood depend on the spleen. Its spread relies on the heart. It is stored in the liver and is transformed by the kidneys. Therefore, pathological changes of the blood are most prominent in the liver, spleen, and kidneys.

Qi and blood vacuity weakness refers to the pathological state of blood vacuity caused by qi deficiency and fatigue. Thus qi vacuity is not able to engender the blood. If blood vacuity lasts a long time, it may lead to the pathological change of qi following the consumption of blood. Hence, qi vacuity and blood deficiency commonly appear together.

The chief symptom of qi vacuity is fatigue. This is often seen in diseases of the digestive system and is accompanied by a sallow, yellow complexion, shortness of breath, disinclination to speak, fatigue of the four limbs, scanty appetite, abdominal distention, loose stools, unreplete stools or lack of force to defecate, a pale, fat tongue, and a vacuous, forceless pulse. Blood deficiency is chiefly characterized by pale white or sallow yellow complexion and pale, lusterless lips and nails. These are commonly seen in patients with chronic loss of blood and are accompanied by heart palpitations, dizziness and vertigo, numbness of the hands and feet, scanty menstruation, delayed menstruation or amenorrhea, a pale tongue, and a fine pulse.

2. QI vacuity & blood stasis

In qi vacuity and blood stasis, qi vacuity results in the movement of the blood being inhibited. In this case, qi vacuity is the root and blood stasis is merely a branch symptom. The chapter titled "The Treatment of Blood *Bi*, Vacuity Taxation & Diseases of the Vessels" of the *Jin Gui Yao Lue (Essentials from the Golden Cabinet)* mentions the blood *bi* pattern. This is the earliest record of the pattern of qi vacuity and blood stasis. Later, physicians in different generations wrote numerous essays on this point. Among them, the essay written by Wang Qing-ren in the Qing Dynasty is the most elaborate. Master Wang points out:

> If the original qi is already vacuous, certainly it cannot reach the blood vessels. Because the vessels are devoid of qi,(the blood) must stop, be retained, and become static.

He emphasized that when the qi is vacuous, there is no force to move the blood. Thus this necessarily produces static blood. Based on this, he advanced the therapeutic principle of using medicinals to supplement the qi and quicken the blood at the same time. Further, he introduced nine formulas for boosting the qi and quickening the blood, including *Bu Yang Huan Wu Tang* (Supplement Yang & Repay the Five [Viscera] Decoction), *Ji Jiu Hui Yang Tang* (Emergency Return Yang Decoction), and *Zhi Xie Tiao Zong Tang* (Stop Diarrhea & Regulate the Center Decoction). These nine formulas are used to treat more than 20 types of diseases and physicians in later generations continue to use them.

The causes leading to blood stasis are numerous, but qi disease leading to static blood is quite common. Qi is the commander of the blood. When qi moves, the blood moves. If qi is vacuous and weak, the propelling force for the circulation of the blood is also reduced. Thus the blood in the vessels will at first flow slowly and later it will become static and stagnant and will produce clots. Thus the pattern of qi vacuity and blood stasis takes form in which there is repletion in the midst of vacuity.

This pattern not only manifests the symptoms of qi vacuity, such as fatigue, shortness of breath, disinclination to talk, weak voice, and feeble breathing but also simultaneously shows the symptoms of static blood, such as aching and pain, swelling and lumps, bluish purple lips and nails, and a purple tongue. One of the clinical points in the discrimination of this pattern is that, after taxation and fatigue, the symptoms of blood stasis become markedly worse. This is because over-taxation aggravates the qi vacuity, rendering it all the more difficult to propel the blood circulation. Therefore, the symptoms of blood stasis are exacerbated. This pattern of qi vacuity and blood stasis is often seen in various geriatric diseases and is also the chief mechanism of senility.

3. Qi stagnation & blood stasis

Qi stagnation and blood stasis refers not only to qi stagnation leading to blood stasis but also to blood stasis leading to qi stagnation. In other words, qi stagnation and blood stasis mutually serve as cause and effect. The pattern of qi stagnation and blood stasis and that of qi vacuity and blood stasis both manifest the symptoms of blood stasis. However, in the former pattern, stasis is due to stagnation and is categorized as a repletion pattern, while in the latter, stasis is caused by vacuity. Thus this pattern is categorized as a root vacuity and branch repletion.

Qi stagnation and blood stasis are gradually formed due to pathological imbalance of the qi mechanism of the viscera and bowels. The commonly observed symptoms have to do with loss of the liver's coursing and discharge. Liver depression leads to qi stagnation. If qi stagnation endures for some time, this leads to the formation of static blood. In addition, if the heart qi loses its harmony, spleen qi does not transport, the lung qi does not diffuse, or the kidney qi does not close, all these will gradually form qi stagnation and blood stasis. Qi stagnation may cause blood stasis, and blood stasis may also cause qi stagnation. For instance, "The Treatise of the Jade Mechanism of the True Treasuries" of the *Su Wen (Simple Questions)* says, "If the vessels and pathways are not open and free-flowing, qi will not come and go." In addition, cold and heat evils may also cause qi stagnation and blood stasis. The chapter in the *Ling Shu (Spiritual Pivot)* titled "*Yong & Ju*" states:

If there is evil cold within the channels and network vessels, blood
will weep (*i.e.*, suffer). Blood weeping leads to its not flowing freely.

This means that cold congeals the qi and blood. The *Yi Lin Gai Cuo
(Correction of Errors in the Medical Forest)* says, "Heat leads to
boiling of the blood and forms stasis." This points out that heat evils
burning internally result in stasis in the blood aspect.

The main symptoms of qi stagnation and blood stasis are chest, lateral
costal, epigastric, and abdominal distention, oppression, aching, and
pain. This pain may be episodic, it may be piercing, and it refuses
pressure. Because this pattern of imbalance is mostly caused by liver
depression, it is often accompanied with emotional tenseness and
agitation. There may be glomus lumps under the lateral costal region.
In women, there may be scanty menstruation, abdominal aching and
pain, or blood clots within the menstruate. The pulse is wiry and the
tongue is purplish. These symptoms are commonly seen in diseases of
the elderly and of middle-aged people, such as chronic gastritis,
cholecystitis, cholelithiasis, chronic hepatitis, neurasthenia, and, in
women, menstrual irregularity.

4. Qi counterflow & blood counterflow

Qi counterflow and blood counterflow refer to confusion and chaos of
the qi mechanism of the viscera and bowels. The qi mechanism
counterflows and does not flow normally. This results in pathological
symptoms of reckless movement of the blood. Under normal conditions
within the human body, the upbearing, downbearing, exiting, and
entering of the qi mechanism of the viscera and bowels proceed
according to a definite rule. For instance, the spleen qi governs
upbearing, while the stomach qi governs downbearing. The liver qi
upbears and emits, while the lung qi depurates and downbears. Heart qi
descends and downbears, while kidney water ascends in a coordinated
manner. This orderly upbearing, downbearing, exiting, and entering is

the basic form of motion in maintaining metabolism of the organism. Qi counterflow is a manifestation of disorder in the upbearing, downbearing, exiting, and entering of the qi mechanism. Qi counterflow may also lead to blood counterflow. "The Treatise on Regulating the Channels" in the *Su Wen (Simple Questions)* states:

> Blood and qi rising together upward lead to great inversion. Inversion leads to sudden death. If qi is restored, one may live again. If it is not restored, there will be death.

This is the earliest record within TCM regarding diseases of the blood vessels in the brain, and its disease mechanism is prompted by the occasion of counterflow of qi, counterflow of blood.

The causes of qi counterflow and blood counterflow are nothing else but the six environmental excesses, the seven emotions, and lack of discipline in eating and drinking. Different of the viscera and bowels are linked to different causes of disease. For instance, counterflow movement of the qi and blood of the lungs is usually due to the six environmental excesses, while counterflow and chaos of the qi and blood of the liver and gallbladder are mostly due to damage by the seven emotions, while loss of normal flow of the spleen and stomach's upbearing and downbearing is mostly due to lack of discipline in eating and drinking.

The pattern of qi counterflow/blood counterflow mostly manifests as diseases of the cerebral blood vessels and in those chiefly symptomized by hemorrhage. Because the physiological functions of the viscera and bowels and the causes of diseases are not the same, the manifestation of qi counterflow and blood counterflow may be divided into those of ascension and those of descension. Qi counterflow and blood counterflow which move upward are commonly due to exuberance of the qi. If the qi has a surplus, fire may occur. Therefore, this is mostly categorized as a repletion pattern. If the liver and stomach qi and blood counterflow upward, this may lead to epistaxis and hematemesis. If the lungs lose their depurating and downbearing and qi and blood counterflow upward, this may lead to hemoptysis. If the kidney qi does not grasp or absorb, ministerial fire may force the qi and blood to become hyperactive above and this may lead to various types of bleeding. If qi and blood counterflow upward to the brain, this may cause wind stroke. If qi and blood counterflow and move downward, this commonly causes qi fall. Qi fall is mostly due to qi vacuity and therefore, this is mostly categorized as a vacuity pattern. For instance, spleen qi and blood may counterflow downward resulting in hemafecia and uterine bleeding. Qi counterflow and blood counterflow leading to the arising of bleeding is summed up in the chapter titled "The Various Arisings of the Hundreds of Diseases" in the *Ling Shu (Spiritual Pivot)* where it states:

> If the yang network vessels are damaged, blood will spill over externally. Spillage of blood externally leads to bleeding. If the yin network vessels are damaged, blood will spill over internally. Internal spillage of blood leads to rear bleeding (*i.e.*, hemafecia).

5. Joining & binding of phlegm & stasis

Joining and binding of phlegm and stasis refers to qi stagnation and phlegm obstruction resulting in the blood's not moving uninhibitedly. If blood stasis stagnates internally, this may also cause stoppage of the fluids and humors and this may also cause the pathological pattern of phlegm and stasis mutually binding together. The *Jing Yue Quan Shu (Complete Writings of Jing-yue)* quotes Wang Jie-zhai as saying:

> Fluids and humors are the surplus of blood. They move outside the vessels and flow freely throughout the entire body. They are like the clear dew of heaven. If blood becomes turbid and qi becomes turbid, they will congeal and gather into phlegm.

Because phlegm is a turbid yin evil, if phlegm is exuberant, it will cause stagnation in the coming and going of the qi. This will gather in and check the channels and vessels. Thus blood will congeal and even more phlegm will be produced. Conversely, static blood obstructing internally may also affect the functioning of the viscera and bowels. This may lead to their loss of command over the spread of fluids and humors with the subsequent engendering of phlegm turbidity. Static blood and phlegm turbidity are both pathological products of metabolism. They mutually engender each other and promote each other's growth. If they stop and stagnate internally in the body, together they may cause the occurence of various pathological changes.

The main symptoms of the joining and binding of phlegm and stasis are dizziness, headache, cough, panting, chest oppression, abdominal distention, heart palpitations, poor memory, excessive dreams, aching and pain of the body and limbs, phlegmy cough, swollen lumps, a purplish tongue with a slimy coating, and a slippery, rapid pulse. These are mostly seen in geriatric diseases, such as coronary heart disease, cardiopulmonary disease, cerebral arteriosclerosis, cervical vertebrae disease, and cancer.

6. Qi not containing the blood

Qi not containing the blood means that, because the qi is vacuous, it is not able to contain and restrain the blood which thus exits causing various types hemorrhagic conditions. Within this pattern, qi vacuity mainly refers to spleen qi vacuity weakness. Inability of qi to contain the blood means, in effect, that the spleen is not able to restrain the blood. Because the spleen qi is insufficient, it has no power to contain the blood which cannot regulate itself. Therefore, it does not circulate along the channels but spills over externally. Spleen qi vacuity may also lead to loss of transportation of the finest essence. Since, in that case, engenderment no longer has a source, blood vacuity becomes even worse.

Qi not containing the blood is mostly due to enduring illness damaging the spleen qi. It may also be caused by loss of regulation in eating and drinking, over-taxation, or too much thought and worry, any of which may damage the spleen qi. Because the spleen qi is vacuous and weak, it loses its power to contain and restrain the blood. Hence the blood spills out of the vessels and thus there appear various types of bleeding disorders.

Qi not containing the blood is characterized by bleeding combined with spleen qi vacuity signs and symptoms. Clinically, there may appear such symptoms as hemorrhage, bloody stool, hematuria, and women's incessant (menstrual) dribbling and dripping. In addition, there may also appear a somber, white, lusterless complexion, spiritual fatigue and lack of strength, shortness of breath, disinclination to talk, and other such signs of spleen qi vacuity weakness. The most important of these are various types of hemorrhagic diseases, such as thrombocytopenic purpura, functional uterine bleeding, and so forth.

7. Blood desertion/qi desertion

Blood desertion/qi desertion refers to the pathological changes associated with the desertion of both the qi and blood due to excessive bleeding. In the chapter titled "Treatment of Blood *Bi*, Vacuity Taxation & Diseases of the Vessels" in the *Jin Gui Yao Lue (Essentials from the Golden Cabinet)*, it says, "If a person's facial color is thin, if there is thirst due to fleeing of blood, if there is sudden wheezing and palpitation, and if the pulse is floating, this means vacuity." "Fleeing of blood" is the pattern of blood desertion. A "floating pulse" means that blood desertion cannot carry the qi. This is thus a manifestation of the qi following blood desertion. "Sudden" denotes that this disease comes all of a sudden, clearly showing that the pattern of blood desertion/qi desertion usually comes suddenly and that the condition of this disease is very critical. Blood desertion/qi desertion and inability of the qi to contain the blood are both patterns of qi and blood dual vacuity.

However, in the former case, along with profuse bleeding, there follows the pattern of qi desertion. Whereas, in the latter case, although the qi is vacuous, there is still no danger of qi desertion or yang desertion. Such bleeding is usually chronic in nature. Thus it is easy to differentiate these two patterns, one from the other.

The blood desertion/qi desertion pattern is mostly caused by sudden bleeding. For instance, if one is injured during a fall, they may bleed incessantly. If a woman suffers from profuse uterine bleeding with loss of an excessive amount of blood, if great anger damages the liver and the patient vomits large amounts of blood, or if they have bloody stools, the disease cannot be cured even though one is treated over a long period. Owing to loss of such a large amount of blood, the original qi cannot adhere anywhere, and so it deserts outwardly, leading to the qi following blood desertion.

The chief clinical manifestations of blood desertion/qi desertion are a somber white complexion, inversion chilling of the four extremities, great sweating which dribbles and drips, and, in severe cases, dizziness inversion (*i.e.*, syncope). The symptoms of external desertion of yang qi often occur simultaneously with the symptom of hemorrhage or may be observed after bleeding. This pattern of imbalance is often seen in shock due to loss of blood.

Static Blood as the Origin of Senility

The two words "*yu xue*" or "static blood" are first seen in the *Jin Gui Yao Lue (Essentials from the Golden Cabinet)* in the chapter titled "Palpitations, Epistaxis, Precipitation of Blood, Chest Fullness & Static Blood Diseases." However, this concept actually originates in the *Nei Jing (Inner Classic)*. The "*e xue*" or "malign blood" mentioned in that book is the earliest record of static blood. Later, Zhang Zhong-jing also referred to this pattern as "retained blood (*liu xue*)", "dry blood (*gan xue*)", and "internal binding (*nei jie*)." Chao Yuan-fang called it "retained blood" and "accumulated blood (*ji xue*)." Zhu Dan-xi called it "dead blood (*si xue*)." Zhang Jing-yue referred to it as "coagulated blood." Wang Ken-tang mentioned it as "foul blood (*kui hui zhi xue*)." Tang Rong-chuan referred to it as "the blood leaving the channel." Thus it can be seen that physicians in different dynasties coined various names for static blood. However, most of these names point to the fact that the formation of static blood is mainly due to loss of harmony of the qi and blood and to the obstruction to its flow and movement. Static blood includes that which is both inside and outside the blood vessels as well as the abnormal composition of the blood.

Uninhibited flow and balance of the qi and blood are signs of the sound health of the organism and also guarantee long life. As the ancients said, "If the blood vessels are open and flowing, diseases cannot obtain engenderment" and "When qi and blood are righteous and even, one's heaven(-decreed) destiny will be long." Conversely, "When qi and blood are not harmonious, hundreds of diseases will transform and be engendered" and these will lead to the senility of the human body. This is because, in that case, blood circulates cyclically and ceaselessly along the vessels throughout the entire body, while qi upbears, downbears, exits, and enters wherever it may reach. It is the circulation of qi and blood which provides the tissues and viscera and bowels of the human body with their required nutrition.

With advancing years, the human body has long been subject to the influences of the seven emotions, six environmental excesses, external injuries, falls and contusions, and various other diseases. Thus there necessarily occurs loss of harmony of qi and blood. Coursing and free flow suffer obstruction, and static blood stops internally. The production and existence of static blood then further inhibits the flow and movement of qi and blood, eveness and balance lose their regulation, and thus the viscera and bowels are not able to obtain their normal nourishment. Phlegm turbidity and various other evils are then engendered internally, and various diseases come in their wake. Then there will appear viscera and bowel vacuity and debility with deficiency and consumption of the essence, qi, and spirit. Because the functions of engenderment and transformation of the qi is decreased, the viscera and bowels cannot perform their physiological functions normally. This then aggravates the loss of balance of the qi and blood and the static blood hidden internally, thus forming a vicious circle and finally leading to senility and death. Therefore we can see that, in the senility of the human body, vacuity is only a symptom, while stasis is its root. Vacuity is the result, while stasis is the cause. The root of human senility consists of static blood.

The above logical arguments are founded on the classics and the statements of famous ancient physicians. However, over a very long period of clinical practice, I have personally observed that, after entering the period of old age, human beings typically manifest marked symptoms of blood stasis. For example, the appearance of skin pigmentation, rough skin, sclerotic opacities, and senile plaques are all typical manifestations of blood stasis. Among the commonly seen geriatric diseases, such as arteriosclerosis, hypertension, coronary heart diseases, wind stroke, senile dementia, prostatic hyperplasia, and diseases of vertebrae in the neck, the cause of these diseases and their clinical manifestations are all related to blood stasis.

In clinical practice, if one simply employs supplementing formulas in their treatment of these diseases, the more one supplements the patient, the more stagnant they become. And the more stagnant they become, the more vacuous they become. However, if we adopt the methods of quickening the blood and transforming stasis, we may get unexpectedly good therapeutic results. This also proves the credibility of the viewpoint that static blood is the origin of senility.

In addition, modern scientific research also confirms that the chief cause of senility is static blood. This mainly manifests in the troubles within the microcirculation, changes in blood rheology, and morphological changes in the blood vessels in different internal organs. After the human body enters the period of old age, troubles in microcirculation impair the function of the transportation and movement of qi and blood as well as the balance of qi and blood. This then disturbs the nerves in the body, the blood vessels, the endocrine system, the immune system, the functions of metabolic manufacture, and the functions of the internal organs. Hence, a series of pathological changes and various signs of senility appear.

All the above arguments, whether theoretical or clinical, prove that the root of senility is loss of balance of the qi and blood and that the fundamental cause of this loss of balance of the qi and blood is static blood.

2

Master Yan's Diagnosis of the Pattern of Static Blood

Based on a combination of our predecessors' experience and clinical surveys of more than 1,239 cases of 50 kinds of disease, it is my opinion that the diagnosis of the pattern of static blood should take the four examinations as its main procedures, while laboratory tests should be used as auxiliary means. These should then be combined with the patient's history. In other words, we should conduct a comprehensive analysis made up of four components: the patient's subjective symptoms, their physical signs, their history, and their laboratory findings. Only then can we make an objective diagnosis.

1. Subjective Symptoms

A. General Symptoms

Fever

Fever occurring in the case of static blood may be of two types: generalized fever and localized fever.

In the case of generalized fever, there may occur a high fever which persists and does not subside. This may be accompanied by hemorrhage, mania and agitation, or local pain. The fever may also be low and lingering. Further, there may be alternating cold and heat, tidal fever in the afternoon, or periodic fever.

In the case of localized fever, the area is red, swollen, aching, and painful. The skin and muscles of the affected area may be burning hot. Localized fever may appear in the areas of the heart and chest, the epigastrium, the lateral costal region, the lower abdomen, the genitalia, the throat, or other such regions. However, in this case, there is no symptom of generalized fever.

Aching & pain

Aching and pain is fixed and immovable. It is confined to a certain spot and refuses pressure. Pain is made worse by pressure. The pain is like a wrenching or the prick of a needle. The pain is difficult to disperse and cannot be eased at once.

Bleeding

This includes hematemesis, hemoptysis, hematuria, hemafecia, uterine bleeding, epistaxis, pyorrhea, bleeding from the flesh, etc. Bleeding may also be due to external injury in turn due to fall or strike. The key points are that the volume of blood is excessive and that the bleeding lasts a long time, is difficult to stop, and tends to occur repeatedly or ceaselessly. The color of the blood may be either dark red or fresh red. The blood usually contains clots. Bleeding may also be accompanied by fever, aching and pain, vexation and agitation, or thirst.

Distention & fullness

The head and eyes, chest and lateral costal regions, epigastrium and abdomen, the lower and upper back, and limbs and body may all have the feelings of distention, fullness, and oppression. The key points are that distention does not decrease, that the feeling of fullness continues for a long time, and that these get worse every day.

Itching

The skin may be affected by itching or it may seems as if worms or ants are crawling beneath the skin and above the muscles. The spot is beyond the reach of one's scratching and the itching occurs spasmodically.

Numbness

The limbs and body may feel numb and insensitive or they may feel as if they were electrified. It is possible for them to lose all sensation and not to be able to know cold from warmth.

Stiffness

The limbs and body may be stiff and awkward and movement is inhibited. The joints cannot bend or stretch. The neck may not be able to turn around. One cannot look up and down easily. They cannot raise or grasp without restriction.

Dry mouth

The mouth may be dry. However, one may rinse it with water but does not wish to drink.

Excessive dreams

One may sleep little but have many dreams which are filled with fright, apprehension, and danger.

Poor memory

There may be heart vexation and insomnia, palpitations and poor memory. One may not be able to rest or their thinking may be confused and chaotic. In extreme cases, one may have raving speech or visual or auditory hallucinations.

B. Symptoms in different systems

Heart system

Heart palpitations, heart pain, spirit orientation confusion and chaos, and mania

Liver/gallbladder system

Emotional depression, excessive suspicion, excessive jealousy, easy vexation, easy agitation, jaundice which does not recede, easy anger, easy violence, lack of constancy in anger and joy

Spleen/stomach system

Epigastric and abdominal aching and pain, distention and fullness, burning heat, dry throat, hiccup, nausea, lack of eating, constipation, and diarrhea

Lung system

Enduring cough, enduring dyspnea, enduring panting (*i.e.* asthma), dry throat, phlegm streaked with red, bloody phlegm, and hemoptysis

Kidney system

Lower abdominal distention, fullness, and tension, turbid urine, urination sometimes astringent and painful, interrupted urination, and scanty urination

2. Physical Signs

Hair

The hair is withered and dry. Its color may be yellowish. It is easily broken and easily falls out.

Face

The color is black or dark. The impression of the face is a darkish complexion. There may be darkish, brown patches or small purple moles on the face. Or the face may be bluish purple, dark red, or blackish.

Eye orbit

The color around the orbit of the eyes is dark and black or dark and lusterless.

Cheeks

The cheeks are flushed red or dark red. There may also be thin, red lines.

Nose

The nose has red scars like acne rosacea.

Lips

The color of the lips is bluish, purple, or dark red.

Chin

The color below the chin is dark.

Eyes

The sclera are static and turbid or have static lines, static spots, static patches, or there may appear patchy lumps. The sclera may also be tinged yellow.

Tongue

The tongue is purple and dark, dark red, or it has static spots and static tumors. The tongue body is emaciated. Its sides may have purplish dark traces. The sinew vessels below the tongue are purple and dark, crooked, distended, full, and exuberant.

Neck

There are greenish blue sinews (*i.e.,* veins) which look angry and distended, full and exuberant in the region of the neck. There may also be tumors, swollen lumps, phlegm nodulations, scrofula, and thin red lines. The blood symptoms on the neck and chest regions may look like the shell of a crab.

Chest

Vacuity inside causes great stirring or throbbing. The skin is dark red or red lines may be seen. The abdominal region is distended and full.

Abdomen

The abdomen is as big as a drum. The navel bulges out. Greenish blue sinews are prominent. One may even feel accumulations and gatherings (*i.e.,* abdominal masses). These ache and are painful when pressed. The lower abdomen is tender, painful, and tense. It may feel hard when pressed.

The lower & upper backs

The vertebrae of the spine of the upper back protrude and are painful when pressed.

The four limbs

The ends of the fingers and toes are enlarged like a pestle. The nails are bluish purple. There is superficial edema of the lower limbs. Locally, the fingers and toes may be a somber white. When pressed, they are as cold as ice. Locally, the feet and toes may be black and severely painful.

Skin

The skin is stiff, stagnant, and hard. It is not elastic when touched. The skin is scaly and dry. Below the skin, there may be static patches, static spots, or the greenish blue sinews below the skin may be prominent. Or there may be swollen lumps, nodulations, black moles, or purplish patches.

3. History

History of enduring illness

Blood stasis often occurs in the case of chronic and recalcitrant diseases which are not healed even after long treatment. Thus it is said, "Enduring disease must have stasis."

Surgical history

After surgery, static blood commonly is retained internally in the body, such as intestinal adhesions and scars.

History of irregular menstruation

There may be a history of dysmenorrhea, amenorrhea, delayed menstruation, scanty menstruation, dark red or purplish red colored blood, and/or blood clots.

History of reproductive abnormality

Male infertility, female infertility, a postpartum lochia which will not stop, postpartum uterine bleeding, postpartum falling of hair, and/or menopause may all be associated with static blood.

Lifestyle history

The patient may be fond of smoking, drinking alcohol, and eating sweet, fatty foods. They may be susceptible to easy anger or fright.

They may have come into contact with pestilential water and contagious qi, etc.

History of external injury

After sustaining external injury, one commonly may have static blood.

Other items in the patient's history

If there is a history of epilepsy, mental diseases, and menopausal syndrome, the patient is usually affected with static blood hidden internally.

4. Laboratory Examination

Examination of blood rheology

In the case of static blood, viscosity of the blood and plasma is typically increased. The sedimentation rate of RBC's is lengthened. The K value in the sedimentation rate is raised. Agglutination of blood cells and the content of fibrinogen are increased. All these are symptoms of static blood.

Examination of nail bed microcirculation

Abnormal capillary loops may be increased. There may be static blood at the top of the loops. The velocity of flow may be reduced. The state of flow may also be abnormal. There may be exudation and bleeding around the capillaries.

Examination of the function of cardiac vessels & dynamics of blood flow

The volume of blood flow may be reduced. In the precordial region, there may be lengthening of PEP and shortening of LVE in the high frequency resistance.

Electrocardiogram & ultrasound examination of cardiac motion

The myocardium may be damaged due to lack of blood. The cardiac ventricle may be hypertrophic. The heart may be enlarged. The valves may be diseased.

Ultrasound examination of the internal organs

The liver and spleen may be enlarged. Hydronephrosis may exists, or a mass may be found in the abdominal cavity.

X-ray examination

There may be inflammation or tumor in the lungs. There may also be a tumor in the abdominal cavity or ulcers, polyps, or diverticula.

Rheoencephalography & electroencephalography

These may reveal cerebral arteriosclerosis, epilepsy, cerebral hematoma, and/or tumor.

Computer-assisted tomography (CAT) & vasography

In the skull and internal organs there may be thrombi, hematoma, and tumors.

Biochemical examination of the blood

There may be hyperlipidemia, chyle in the serum, and high bilirubin.

Routine examination of the blood

Erythrocytes, leukocytes, and platelets may be increased.

Other Items

There may be lupus cells, positive rheumatoid factors, and antis-treptolysin O in the blood. Blood sedimentation may be accelerated, and albumin may be increased.

The basis for concluding a diagnosis of static blood pattern may be made from a combination of the above-mentioned four categories, namely, subjective symptoms, bodily signs, history, and laboratory findings. Clinically, if there are more than four criteria within any two of these categories, one may diagnose the disease as manifesting a pattern of static blood.

3

The Relationship Between the Symptoms of Senility & Static Blood

The key characteristic of senility is that, with advancing years, there is general degeneration and impediment in the organic functioning of the various viscera and bowels. The chief difference between senility and disease is that the functional degeneration of the viscera and bowels caused by diseases is only confined to certain of the viscera and bowels, while that caused by senility involves almost all the organs in the body. This is the result of blood stasis on the metabolic processes of the organism.

Changes in the essence spirit & spirit orientation

As the elderly get ever older, poor memory may occur and the incidence of essence spirit abnormalities, diminished intelligence, and dementia gradually rises. This is one of the important manifestations of senility.

In TCM it is thought that "Spirit is the nature of blood and qi." Only when qi and blood are full and exuberant can one's spirit orientation be clear and distinct and one's spirit be full and abundant. "The Treatise on the Eight Righteous Spirit Brilliances" in the *Su Wen (Simple Questions)* says, "Blood and qi are a human's spirit." The chapter titled "Average People Ceasing Grain" in the *Ling Shu (Spiritual Pivot)* says, "When the blood vessels are harmonious and uninhibited, the essence spirit can then abide there." These sayings point out the fact that blood, qi, and spirit orientation are all closely related. Owing to long harassment by the seven emotions, if the emotions of the elderly are excessively disturbed, if one is troubled by thought, irritation, and anger, or if overtaxation damages the heart and spleen, then this will necessarily affect the uninhibited flow of blood and will cause loss of harmony of the qi and blood. Blood stasis will stop internally and there will be loss of nourishment in the brain. Thus there will occur poor memory and diminished intelligence and other such changes in one's spirit orientation. If severe, there may even be dementia and insanity.

According to modern research, senile dementia refers to serious degeneration in perception, memory, and the ability to think abstractly and inventively. This occurs in people over 60 years of age due to organic changes in their cerebrum or due to sustained metabolic damage. Further, this condition is related to disorders in the cerebral circulation and lack of blood in the whole brain. In addition, decrease in the volume of blood flowing in the whole brain is directly proportional to the severity of this dementia.

In the ancient literature of Chinese medicine, there are numerous records of blood stasis causing changes in the essence spirit and spirit orientation. For instance, the *Shang Han Lun (Treatise on Damage due to Cold)* says, "One who is oblivious must have stored blood." Tang Rong-chuan, in his *Xue Zheng Lun (Treatise on Bleeding Patterns)* says, "Whoever's heart has static blood will also be affected by poor memory" and "Anyone with loss of blood who suddenly has poor memory has static blood." In the *Yi Lin Gai Cuo (Corrections of Mistakes in the Medical Forest)* it is recorded, "Qi and blood may congeal and stagnate the brain qi." All these sayings clearly show that changes in the essence spirit and spirit orientation in the elderly are connected with blood stasis.

Heart palpitations, racing heart & heart pain

Heart palpitations and racing heart are important manifestations of senility of the circulatory system. Owing to degeneration in the retentive ability of old peoples' hearts, they are usually affected by various heart diseases. Heart palpitations and racing heart are both manifestations of various cardiac diseases.

According to TCM, heart palpitations, racing heart, and heart pain are closely related to blood stasis. The chapter titled "Channels & Vessels" in the *Ling Shu (Spiritual Pivot)* states:

> If the hand *shao yin* qi is exhausted, the vessels will not be open. If the vessels are not open, the blood will not flow.

This is because:

> The heart is *tai yang* within yang. If *tai yang* does not grow, then heart qi internally will be fearful.

"Fearful" means empty and vacuous. Because the qi of heart yang is vacuous, it has no strength to stir or throb and this may lead to blood stasis and *bi* obstruction in the heart vessels. Pathologically, blood stasis is similar to weakened myocardiac contractile force, coronary arteriosclerosis, and lack of blood and oxygen in the myocardium. The vessels are the mansion of the blood, and the heart, vessels, and blood are all mutually connected. If the condition of the heart, blood, and vessels is normal, this ensures that the transportation of blood is uninhibited and free-flowing. If the heart qi's power of propulsion has no force, if the heart loses its nourishing blood, or if the vessels and network vessels are blocked and obstructed, then blood flow will be inhibited and the symptoms of heart palpitations, racing heart, and, if severe, heart pain will appear.

Heart palpitations and racing heart in the elderly commonly appear in the following two guises:

1) Lack of force of heart qi's power of propulsion

The ability of the heart to transport and move the blood flow depends upon the function of the yang qi within the heart. "The Treatise on the Signs of Qi in Average People" in the *Su Wen (Simple Questions)* refers to this qi as "the qi of the blood vessels treasured by the heart." "The

Treatise on the Vessels & the Finest Essence" in the *Su Wen (Simple Questions)* states:

> The vessels (or in this case the pulse) is the mansion of the blood. If it is long, qi is normal. If it is short, qi is diseased...If it is regularly interrupted, qi is debilitated. If it is fine, qi is scanty. If it is choppy, there is heart pain.

This points out that long pulse is the manifestation of sufficient qi, while short, regularly interrupted, and fine pulses are manifestations of heart qi insufficiency. This is finds its expression in a lack of force to propel the blood vessels. Because the elderly person's heart qi is vacuous and weak, therefore their blood vessels are static and stagnant. Hence a regularly interrupted pulse and heart pain may be seen.

2) Static blood obstructing and stagnating in the heart vessels

The heart depends on blood for its nourishment, while the blood relies on qi for its propulsion. Because the elderly are incessantly subjected to external evils, their lung qi is consumed and damaged. Thus their qi is vacuous, while their blood is static. Or, if they have long been affected by *bi* patterns "internally housed in the heart", this may also lead to inhibition of the flow of heart blood. In that case, stasis may obstruct the vessels and network vessels and it may become apparent that blood is not nourishing the heart. Thus the symptoms of heart palpitations, racing heart, and cyanosis may appear.

Wind stroke & hemiplegia

The *Dong Yuan Shi Shu (Ten Books of Dong-yuan)* states:

> Wind stroke is the greatest of the hundreds of diseases. It is caused by blockage of the qi and blood which then does not move. It is the most serious disease.

Wind stroke is a common cause of death in the elderly, and physicians in different generations have attached importance to the relationship between wind stroke and static blood. The *Nei Jing (Inner Classic)* refers to it as "vertex disease", "mean inversion", and "great inversion." "The Treatise on Engendering Qi Communicating with Heaven" in the *Su Wen (Simple Questions)* says, "Great anger makes the form qi exhausted, while blood flows upward, thus causing mean inversion." "The Treatise on Regulating the Channels" says, "Blood and qi both flow upward leading to great inversion." This clearly explains that the location of this disease is in the head and that its main disease mechanism is the upward flow of blood. The pattern of wind stroke may not only manifest symptoms of unconsciousness, wry mouth, and inability to speak, but it may also manifest hemiplegia and inability to use the limbs. The *Sheng Ji Zong Lu (General Collection for Holy Relief)* states:

> As regards wind stroke, if the tongue is stiff and the patient cannot speak, this is because the spleen and stomach vessels and network vessels grasp the throat and tongue where the heart qi flows. Wind and evil guests struggle. Therefore the qi in the vessels is blocked, hindered, and inhibited. The tongue is stiff and cannot roll freely, thus handicapping one's voice and speech.

"Abstruse Mechanisms & Origins of Disease" in the *Su Wen (Simple Questions)* says, "When one has been struck, qi and blood do not flow freely and one side withers." The *Zheng Yin Mai Zhi (Patterns, Causes, Pulses & Treatment)* states:

> The cause of hemiplegia may be qi congelation of qi and blood stagnation. Or there may be stomach heat engendering phlegm. This flows into the channel tunnels and cuts off their pathways. Thus qi and blood cannot move forward and backward.

Hence it is apparent that the relationship of wind stroke to static blood and phlegm obstruction is truly indisputable.

Cough & asthma

Cough and asthma are common diseases in the elderly. This is related to the fact that the elasticity of old peoples' lungs is decreased. This decrease of elasticity is accompanied by diminished function of breathing and by chronic diseases of the respiratory system. Long-standing cough and shortness of breath are often accompanied by barrel chest or senile emphysema and cyanosis. All these are closely related to phlegm obstruction and blood stasis. In his *Xue Zheng Lun (Treatise on Bleeding Patterns)*, Tang Rong-chuan points out:

> Blood stasis assails the lungs and cough, counterflow, and panting occur. The path of qi in the human body must have congestion and stagnation. If there is blood stasis internally, this obstructs and hinders the path of qi which cannot then obtain upbearing and downbearing but congests and causes cough.

The *Dan Xi Xin Fa (Dan-xi's Heart Methods)* also states:

> When the lungs are distended, there is cough. One turns to the left or right, but cannot go to sleep. This is because phlegm mixed with stasis hinders the qi and causes diseases.

Cough and asthma in the elderly start first from the lungs and later affect the heart. Because the heart rules the construction and blood and the lungs face the hundreds of vessels, they help the heart to move the blood vessels. All the blood in the entire body passes through the blood vessels and gathers in the lungs where the turbid qi is exhaled while the clear qi is absorbed. Thus it is able to spread and scatter to the entire body. Therefore, if lung disease is advanced, lung qi will necessarily be consumed and phlegm turbidity will be engendered internally. The heart and lungs will both become diseased. Phlegm turbidity will obstruct internally and affect the transportation and movement of blood. The vessels and network vessels will become static and obstructed and that will eventually involve the heart. For instance, in the latter stages of cough and asthma, one may often see heart palpitations, chest oppression, cyanotic lips, prominent greenish blue sinews, and a bound or regularly irregular pulse. If this has endured for some time, static blood will transform into water and produce water swelling or edema. According to modern research, senile chronic bronchitis, emphysema, and pulmonary heart disease all involve pathological changes resulting from phlegm obstruction and blood stasis. If medicinals are used to eliminate phlegm and transform stasis, this produces good therapeutic effects.

Dizziness, vertigo & scant sleep

Old people frequently experience dizziness, vertigo, and scant sleep. The channels and vessels, qi and blood of old people decline every day. The blood vessels' transportation and movement is inhibited. Stasis obstructs the clear portals. Qi and blood are not able to ascend to nourish the head and eyes. This may manifest as dizziness, vertigo, and scant sleep. In the *Yi Deng Xu Yan (Keeping the Flame of the Lamp of Medicine Lit)*, Pan Ji in the Qing Dynasty said:

> All yang moves upward to the head. Clear yang moves upward to the eyes. If blood dies, the vessels congeal and weep. If the vessels congeal and weep, the force of flowing upward will become thin. If it becomes thin, there will be vacuity above and dizziness and vertigo will be engendered.

The *Zhang Shi Yi Tong (Master Zhang's Medical Knowledge)* says, "If within the chest the blood is dead, there will be pain and dizziness." The *Yi Lin Gai Cuo (Corrections of Mistakes in the Medical Forest)* says, "If at night while asleep there are excessive dreams, this is static blood." All these cites clearly explain the disease mechanism at work in this condition.

Modern research confirms that most of the elderly are affected by cerebral arteriosclerosis, diseases in the vertebrae of the neck, and an insufficient supply of blood in the arteries at the base of the vertebrae. All these cause a decrease in the volume of blood flowing into the brain.

The tissues in the brain thus lack blood and oxygen and hence give rise to dizziness, vertigo, and scant sleep. If an effective method for dilating the blood vessels and increasing the volume of blood flowing to the brain and the amount of oxygen in the blood is adopted, then dizziness may be relieved. The condition of sleep will be improved, and the senility of cerebral cells may be delayed.

White hair & falling hair

White or grey hair is an important physical characteristic of senility. In his essay, "Treatise on Balance (*Lun Heng*)", Wang Chong points out:

> When a person's body is old, their skin and hair change color. When one is young, their hair is black. When they are old, it becomes white.

The chapter titled "Channels & Vessels" in the *Ling Shu (Spiritual Pivot)* states:

> If the hand *shao yin* qi is exhausted, then the vessels will not be open. The blood will not flow freely. If the blood does not flow, the color of the hair will not be shiny.

The *Xue Zheng Lun (Treatise on Bleeding Patterns)* says, "If there is static blood in the upper burner, the hair will shed and will not grow." The *Yi Lin Gai Cuo (Correction of Mistakes in the Medical Forest)* also states:

> Blood stasis between the skin and the interior, the internal and the external may obstruct and hinder the vessels and network vessels. Fresh blood is thus not able to nourish the hair. Therefore, the hair falls out and sheds. If there is no disease but the hair falls out, this is also static blood.

Thus it can be seen that blood stasis is an important cause of baldness and white hair.

Diminished visual power & auditory power

From ancient times, diminished visual and auditory power have been important criteria for estimating the degree of one's senility. Changes in the visual power of the aged essentially means decline in the eyesight, blindness, corneal diseases, and senile cataracts or arcus senilis, while changes in auditory power mainly refer to tinnitus and deafness.

According to TCM, decline in eyesight and hearing in the elderly is chiefly caused by loss of balance of the qi and blood in the viscera and bowels, by static blood stopping internally, and by inability of liver/-kidney essence and blood to ascend and construct the empty portals. The *Nei Jing (Inner Classic)* says, "When the eyes obtain blood, they can see." Blood is able to moisten the channels and network vessels and the viscera and bowels. It nourishes the sinews and bones, fills the entire body, and, when the eyes get it, they are shaded. Therefore, it is appropriate that blood flows freely and it is not appropriate for it to become static and stagnant. If static blood obstructs and hinders or essence and blood do not rise to the empty portals, then the eyes will not be clear. The *Huang Han Yi Xue (The Study of Imperial Han Medicine)* also says, "If there are the above-mentioned patches and spots or purple and blue colors on the conjunctiva, this also proves the pattern of blood stasis."

Modern research confirms that, in the ocular fundus of elderly eyes which have undergone senile degenerative changes, the superficial blood vessels become thin, the color of the retina becomes dark, there may be large white patches or atrophic patches, and the color of the optic nerve becomes light. All these are phenomena associated with insufficient supply of blood. This coincides with the theory of blood stasis in TCM. In treating the above conditions, if one uses quickening the blood and transforming stasis formulas so that the qi and blood move uninhibitedly, then the power of the vision may be restored.

In terms of diminished auditory power, although this has something to do with the kidney function, yet it is also closely connected to static blood. *Yi Lin Gai Cuo (Corrections of Mistakes in the Medical Forest)* states:

> In the ear, there is a small tube opening to the brain. If outside this tube there is static blood which presses and closes this tube, the ears will become deaf.

At the same time, the heart governs all the blood vessels in the body. For hearing to be normal, their form must be filled with a combination of qi and blood. If qi and blood are empty and vacuous within the vessels and are not able to ascend and construct or if qi and blood transportation and movement is inhibited, this may also cause diminished hearing or tinnitus. As the chapter titled "Forms of Disease of Evil Qi in the Viscera & Bowels" in the *Ling Shu (Spiritual Pivot)* says, "If the heart pulse is minute and choppy, this will produce tinnitus."

Senile patches & scaly, dry skin

The brown spots on the skin of the face, hands, and upper back are called *lao nian ban* or old age patches and *shou ban*, longevity patches. Investigation confirms that the incidence of these brown patches on the skin increases with age. Seventy-five percent of people aged 60-79 have them, while 89% of those aged 80-90 have them. Moreover, if these brown patches on the skin spread widely, then senility is severe. Thus we may see that old age patches are universally accepted as a criterion for determining the senility of the organism. At the same time, old peoples' skin also becomes rough, inelastic, and pigmented darkly. TCM refers to this as scaly, dry skin, and it is a typical symptom of static blood.

Scaly, dry skin is caused by vacuity taxation blood stasis, in which case there is dry blood internally. Because the elderly are affected by blood stasis, fresh blood is not engendered, while vanquished blood accumulates. Therefore, the skin loses its moistening and nourishment and becomes rough. In addition, superfluous substance and neoplastic tissue may grow. The *Yi Meng Fa Lu (Law in Medical Science)* states:

> The skin is scaly, dry. The face and eyes become dark and emaciated. One cannot drink or eat. All the constructive blood becomes static and accumulates within. This appears on the skin of the face and eyes.

The *Zhu Bing Yuan Hou Lun (Treatise on the Cause & Symptoms of Various Diseases)* says that scaly, dry skin is due to "blood and qi glomus and astringency so that moisture cannot flow freely to the skin." Scaly, dry skin is now regarded as an important criterion for diagnosing static blood.

Prominent greenish blue sinews & cyanosis

The exposure of prominent greenish blue sinews (*i.e.,* veins) in the elderly refers to various varicose phenomena, such as sublingual varices and varicosities on the lower limbs or the abdominal wall as well as dilation of capillaries on the nail bed and cheeks. In some old people, one may also see cyanosis. This may appear on their lips and at tips of their extremities.

As regards the subject of static blood and its relationship to the exposure of prominent greenish blue sinews and cyanosis, there have been many essays written on this subject, both ancient and modern. For instance, the *Gu Jin Yi Jian (The Mirror of Ancient & Modern Medicine)* says, "As regards the pattern of exposure of greenish blue sinews, its source is qi counterflow and blood not moving". The *Yi Xue Zheng Chuan (The True Understanding of Medical Theory)* states:

> If blood is quickened, it will be red. If blood congeals, it will be black. If the nails are black, then blood has congealed and does not scatter.

The *Jin Gui Yao Lue (Essential Prescriptions from the Golden Chamber)* says, "If the lips are atrophic and the tongue becomes greenish blue, the mouth is not being constructed (*i.e.*, being nourished by construction and blood)." The *Yi Lin Gai Cuo (Corrections of Mistakes of the Medical Forest)* says even more clearly:

> Prominent greenish blue sinews are not sinews. What appears on the skin is the blood vessels. Greenish blue vessels show that there is stasis internally.

Because of decrease in elasticity of the vessels in the elderly, the heart qi is deficient and debilitated. The blood does not move uninhibitedly. Static blood stops internally. The vessels and network vessels shrink. Therefore, greenish blue sinews appear prominently.

In recent years, members of the TCM circle have made relatively detailed observations of the static sinews below the tongue in the elderly and have come to regard these as an important means of diagnosing static blood. Through research it has been discovered that the protrusion of the veins below the tongue is directly proportional to the increase in age. The increase in the diameter of the trunk of the veins below the tongue and their morphological changes are particularly pronounced in people from 60-65 years of age. This shows that static veins below the tongue are not only a sign of aging but also are a criterion for estimating and determining the exuberance or decline of the viscera and bowels in the elderly.

Fatigue & lack of appetite

With advancing age, a person's activities gradually decrease. They are easily fatigued and this is often accompanied by loss of appetite and atrophy of the muscles of the four limbs. According to TCM, the appearance of these symptoms is due to spleen vacuity since the spleen governs the muscles of the whole body. The four limbs of the human body require spleen qi to transport and spread construction and nourishment, thus enabling the maintenance of normal physiological activities. If construction and nourishment are sufficient, then the muscles and flesh of the four limbs are full and they are dexterous and forceful. If the spleen loses its fortification and transportation, then clear yang will not spread. This insufficiency of construction and nourishment will cause atrophy of the muscles and flesh and lassitude and lack of strength of the four limbs. Thus "The Treatise on *Tai Yang & Yang Ming*" in the *Su Wen (Simple Questions)* states:

> The four limbs receive qi from the stomach as a boon, but the qi is not obtained by the channels. This must be due to the spleen, for it can obtain such a boon. If the spleen is diseased and not able to produce the stomach's movement of the fluids and humors, the four limbs cannot obtain the boon of water and grain qi. Therefore, the qi becomes debilitated every day. The vessel pathways are inhibited, and the sinews and bones, muscles and flesh have no qi to engender them. Thus they cannot function well.

By this we may see that spleen qi debility and stasis and obstruction of the vessels and pathways are related to the non-functioning of the four limbs.

Water swelling & dribbling urinary block

Owing to decline in the function of their heart and kidneys and to trouble in the circulation of their veins, edema of the lower limbs is frequently observed in the elderly. According to TCM, the formation of water swelling has to do with loss of regulation of the lungs, spleen, and kidneys. If the lungs are diseased, they will not be able to open and regulate the water passageways. If the spleen is diseased, it will not be able to transport and transform the water dampness. If the kidneys are diseased, qi transformation will be inhibited. If one inquires into the cause of all this, it is all due to inhibition of the water passageways, and this is closely related to static blood. In his *Xue Zheng Lun (Treatise on*

Bleeding Patterns), Tang Rong-chuan points out, "Static blood may transform into water and also produce water swelling." Because the elderly's viscera and bowel function is diminished, their qi is vacuous and lacks propulsive power. The transportation and movement of the blood flow is inhibited. Stasis obstructs the water passageways, and water dampness spills over internally into the muscles and skin. Thus water swelling appears.

Old peoples' urination is also inhibited. This is mainly manifest as retention of urine. This retention is mostly caused by kidney qi deficiency and detriment and by static blood obstructing and stagnating in urinary tract. The *Xue Zheng Lun (Treatise on Blood Patterns)* says, "If there is blood stasis in the lower burner, there is pain below the lumbar region and the lower abdomen and lateral costal regions will be distended and full." In treating prostatic hyperplasia, supplementing the kidneys *and* quickening the blood produces better therapeutic effect.

Diminished sexual function

Diminished sexual function mainly refers to impotence in men and amenorrhea in women. Impotence is a common disease in men over 60 years of age. Impotence in the elderly is a natural physiological phenomenon and reflects the senility of the human body. As "The Great Treatise on the Resonances & Appearances of Yin & Yang" in the *Su Wen (Simple Questions)* says, "At 60 years of age, impotence occurs, qi is greatly debilitated, and the nine portals are inhibited."

For a long time, members of the medical circle have thought that impotence is caused by kidney vacuity. In fact, impotence has a close relationship with static blood. This is because the kidneys rule the treasuring of essence, while the liver governs coursing and discharge. The channels and vessels of the liver surround the genitals. It is the normal functioning of the liver's coursing and discharge which enables to the closing and treasuring of the kidneys. In addition, essence and blood have a common source and produce each other. Therefore, if coursing and discharge by the liver lose their normalcy, then the qi and blood will not move uninhibitedly. Thus stasis will obstruct the vessels of the yin (*i.e.*, genitalia), and this may lead to impotence. Hence, marked effects may be obtained if one treats impotence by quickening the blood and transforming stasis.

Amenorrhea is also closely related to static blood. The *Yi Xue Ru Men (Entering the Gate of the Study of Medicine)* states:

> Hundreds of diseases in the channels are caused by blood stagnation and withering. In women, blood production rules. When heaven's true qi is downborne, the *tian gui* arrives. When the kidney qi is whole and exuberant, blood vessels flow and move. Hence (the menstrual discharge) is observed once every 3 times 10 days, just like the waxing and waning of the moon.

Owing to vacuity and debility of the *chong* and *ren* in older women, the qi and blood are inhibited and stasis obstructs the *bao mai*. The *bao gong* thus loses its nourishment, for if stasis lasts long, nourishment will surely decline. If the constructive and the blood become scanty, amenorrhea will occur. Therefore, one should not neglect the factor of static blood.

Muscle & skin numbness, limb and body aching & pain

Muscle and skin numbness and limb and body aching and pain belong to the category of blood *bi*. "The Treatise on *Bi*" in the *Su Wen (Simple Questions)* says, "If there is *bi* in the vessels, blood will congeal and does not flow." The *Di Yu Sui Bi (Notes on the Study of Medicine)* says, "Blood in the channels and network vessels may be divided into aching and pain and numbness." Owing to the daily decline in the qi and blood of the elderlys' channels and vessels, the blood vessels' transportation and movement is inhibited. The muscles and skin and the sinews and bones lose their nourishment. Hence numbness of the muscles and skin and aching and pain of the limbs and body appear. These sensations may occur repeatedly, or they may linger endlessly. Further, they may spread over the entire body. Ye Tian-shi said, "Enduring diseases enter the network vessels." Because the elderlys' qi and blood transportation and movement are inhibited, within the blood network vessels there is stasis and congelation. If this is not eliminated, freshly engendered blood will not be able to flow freely and eventually the original qi will not be able to be restored.

4

Quickening the Blood & Regulating the Qi as an Effective Method for Combating Senility

Because diseases of the qi and blood reflect, as a whole, the loss of normalcy of the viscera and bowels and organic senility, one may treat various diseases and patterns of imbalance of the viscera and bowels based on the principles of regulating and harmonizing the qi and blood, thereby restoring health and delaying senility. Thus different diseases may be effectively treated using a single method. As "The Treatise on the Three Parts & Nine Symptoms" in the *Su Wen (Simple Questions)* states:

> First it is necessary to determine whether the body is fat or thin so as to regulate the vacuity and repletion of qi. If there is repletion, it should be drained. If there is vacuity, it should be supplemented. First it is necessary to empty the blood vessels and afterwards regulate (the qi. Even) without inquiring into the disease, one should expect to get balance.

The chapter titled "*Yong & Ju*" in the *Ling Shu (Spiritual Pivot)* also says, "Once the blood and qi are regulated, then the form qi can be preserved."

"Expecting to get balance" means that, through regulation and discipline of the qi and blood, the qi and blood which were in a state of imbalance may come to a new state of balance, thus ensuring a ceaseless supply of enriching and nourishing qi and blood to the viscera and bowels, rectifying the vacuity and debility of the viscera and bowels, and promoting the balance and coordination of their physiological function. This will then place the human body in a dynamic state of balance so that the person in question may become an average (literally level or healthy) human being.

In treating disease, TCM usually follows the principle of "leveling yin and secreting yang", thinking that the occurrence of any disease is completely due to loss of regulation of yin and yang. Therefore, there is the theory that, "One should scrutinize the existence of yin and yang and regulate them so as to get balance." Because qi and blood are the main material bases of yin and yang in the human body, so "The Great Treatise on the Supreme Truth" in the *Su Wen (Simple Questions)* states:

> If one observes the *dao* just like the law, then ten thousand deeds, ten thousand completions. Qi and blood will be righteous and level, and one's heaven(-decreed) destiny will be long.

This is because the uninhibited and free flow of qi and blood balance yin and yang, make disease disappear, and preserve one's health and longevity.

TCM lays special emphasis on the function of regulating, coursing, and freeing the flow of qi and blood. Wang Qing-ren of the Qing Dynasty said:

> The essential secret of treating disease is clearly knowing the qi and blood. Be it external evil or internal damage, it is essential to know that first disease damages a person's substance. It is not able to damage the viscera and bowels, it is not able to damage the sinews and bones. Rather it damages nothing other than their qi and blood.

Because qi and blood belong to the same category, therefore the "regulating the qi" or "regulating the channels" mentioned in the *Nei*

Jing (Inner Classic) means the method of regulating both the qi and blood. As "The Great Treatise on the Supreme Truth" in the *Su Wen (Simple Questions)* points out:

> The way to regulate qi is necessarily to distinguish between yin and yang, to determine the middle and the exterior, and to keep their respective regions. Internal (disease) should be treated internally. External (diseases) should be treated externally. In mild cases, simply regulate (the qi) and there will be levelness or calm. If there is exuberance, it should be seized by force. Sweat should be precipitated, cold, heat, warmth, and coolness should be debilitated. According to the condition of the case, if one observes this *dao* like law, then ten thousand deeds, ten thousand completions. Qi and blood will be righteous and level and one's heaven(-decreed) destiny will be long.

Again it says:

> Acridity emits and sweetness scatters yang, while sour and bitter open and discharge yin. The salty flavor opens and discharges yin, while the bland flavor percolates and discharges yang. Thus the six flavors either restrain or scatter. They may be mild or they may be drastic, drying or moistening, softening or hardening. Everywhere (the qi) should be disinhibited and moved, for the regulation of qi results in levelness (*i.e.*, normal health).

Besides regulating and disciplining the qi and blood from outside by using medicinal substances, ancient physicians also used the methods of acupuncture and moxibustion to regulate and disinhibit the qi and blood. For instance, the chapter titled "Nine Needles & Twelve Causes" in the *Ling Shu (Spiritual Pivot)* says, "Use a minute needle to free the flow of the vessels, regulate the qi and blood, and meet the point where counterflow and normal flow issue." The chapter titled "Explanation of the Small Needle" in the *Ling Shu (Spiritual Pivot)* further states:

counterflow and normal flow issue." The chapter titled "Explanation of the Small Needle" in the *Ling Shu (Spiritual Pivot)* further states:

> In general, take care of the form. This means taking care of the method of needling. Moreover, take care of the spirit. Take care whether a person's qi and blood have a surplus or are insufficient.

Through selecting points along the channels and needling them to obtain the qi, one may course and free the flow of qi and blood in the channels and network vessels. Thus various diseases may be cured and the person may obtain good health.

In short, "Qi is the chief of the hundreds of diseases" and "Blood is the fetus of the hundreds of diseases." Qi and blood running counter to reason and acting perversely are the guiding principle of the hundreds of diseases. Thus, "If qi is free flowing and blood is quickened, then there is nothing which cannot be eliminated." "Balancing yin and yang" and "regulating and smoothing the qi and blood" means the treating of disease. Therefore, it is my belief that in treating and preventing disease, combating senility and increasing longevity, we should take the theory of qi and blood as our theoretical basis. We should emphasize the word "balance." If we take the word "balance" into account, then, just as it is said, "Once the headrope of a fishing net is pulled in", we will easily get the real effect.

5

The Clinical Application of the Balancing Method

The clinical application of the balancing method in the treatment of senility does not simply mean piling up medicinals which quicken the blood and transform stasis. Instead, there are strict rules guiding its implementation in a rational manner. In applying this method, one should take care not to depart from the basic spirit of pattern discrimination and treatment in TCM. One must first clearly know the cause and mechanism of the disease at hand. Then one may determine the treatment principles, select the appropriate formula, and use the appropriate medicinals. Only thus will one's therapeutic results increase.

Although medicinals which quicken the blood and transform and dispel stasis all share the common characteristics of freeing and disinhibiting the blood vessels and eliminating static blood, they also have their different individual characteristics, such as cooling the blood, stopping bleeding, opening the network vessels, moving the qi, precipitating water, and nourishing the blood. In addition, they each have their own nature. For instance, they may be cold, hot, warm, or cool. Therefore, when applying medicinals in clinical practice, one should select medicinals for quickening the blood and transforming stasis which correspond to the patient's pattern discrimination. Then one can expect to obtain satisfactory results. Based on clinical experience, the balancing method is composed of ten methods of prescribing ingredients.

1. Rectifying the qi & transforming stasis method

When used together, medicinals which rectify the qi and medicinals which quicken the blood are indicated for the treatment of tension, distension, and pain in the chest and lateral costal regions, lack of constancy of joy and anger, or if one's behavior is contrary. Such kinds of patterns are often caused by liver qi depression and accumulation. The commonly used formulas are *Xue Fu Zhu Yu Tang* (Blood Mansion Dispel Stasis Decoction), *Ge Xia Zhu Yu Tang* (Below the Diaphragm Dispel Stasis Decoction), and *Fu Yuan Huo Xue Tang* (Restore the Origin & Quicken the Blood Decoction). This method is suitable for functional nervous diseases, chronic colitis, infertility, hysteria, and coronary heart disease as well as diseases of the hepatic and biliary systems.

Treatment principles: Course & discharge the liver qi, quicken the blood and transform stasis

Rx: Radix Bupleuri (*Chai Hu*), 9g, Radix Ligustici Wallichii (*Chuan Xiong*), 9g, Rhizoma Cyperi Rotundi (*Xiang Fu*), 9g, Fructus Citri Seu Ponciri (*Zhi Qiao*), 5g, Radix Platycodi Grandiflori (*Jie Geng*), 5g, Radix Achyranthis Bidentatae (*Niu Xi*), 5g, Flos Carthami Tinctorii (*Hong Hua*), 9g, Semen Pruni Persicae (*Tao Ren*), 9g, Radix Salviae Miltiorrhizae (*Dan Shen*), 15g

Indications: Chest and lateral costal aching and pain, insomnia, excessive dreams, emotional depression, excessive suspicion, and other such abnormal changes in one's emotions.

Formula rationale: The liver rules coursing and discharge. If one desires for the qi and blood to be level and balanced, then first seek the coursing and discharge of the liver qi. Therefore, Bupleurum and Cyperus course and discharge the liver qi. Ligusticum, Carthamus, Persica, and Salvia quicken the blood and transform phlegm and are the heart kernel of this formula. These are assisted by Platycodon, Citrus, and Achyranthes which course and disinhibit the qi and blood in the upper, middle, and lower parts, thus spreading the actions of this formula of balancing yin and yang and regulating the qi and quickening the blood throughout the entire body.

2. Scattering cold & quickening the blood method

When used together, warming the interior medicinals and quickening the blood medicinals are indicated for chest, lateral costal, epigastric, and abdominal pain as well as *bi* pain of the four limbs. This pain may be very severe. The tongue is bluish and its coating is white. In this case, cold evils have caused stasis in the channels and vessels and women's uterine diseases are commonly seen. For stasis in the channels and vessels, use *Yang He Tang* (Harmonize Yang Decoction), *Dang Gui Si Ni Tang* (Dang Gui Four Counterflows Decoction), and *Wu Yu Sheng Jiang Tang* (Evodia & Fresh Ginger Decoction). If cold has congealed in the uterus, then use *Sheng Hua Tang* (Engendering & Transforming Decoction). This method may be used with various gynecological diseases, such as dysmenorrhea, infertility, adnexitis, and ectopic pregnancy. It is also indicated for pain in the heart and abdomen, including angina pectoris, obstructive pain, porphyria, and Raynaud's disease.

Treatment principles: Warm, scatter, and transform congelation, dispel stasis and stop pain

Rx: Radix Bupleuri (*Chai Hu*), 6g, Cortex Cinnamomi (*Guan Gui*), 5g, Feces Trogopterori Seu Pteromi (*Wu Ling Zhi*), 9g, uncooked Pollen Typhae (*Pu Huang*), 9g, Rhizoma Corydalis Yanhusuo (*Yan Hu Suo*), 9g, Resina Myrrhae (*Mo Yao*), 4.5g, dry Rhizoma Zingiberis (*Gan Jiang*), 2.4g, Radix Ligustici Wallichii (*Chuan Xiong*), 9g, Flos Caryophylli (*Gong Ding Xiang*), 3g

Indications: Chilly pain in the chest and abdomen, women's menstrual pain, female infertility

Formula rationale: Cold residing in the blood results in congelation. Therefore, treatment should consist of both warming and eliminating stasis. In this formula, Pollen Typhae, Feces Trogopterori, Ligusticum, and Myrrh, which quicken the blood, are the sovereigns. The ministers are Cinnamon, dry Ginger, and Cloves for warming and transporting. The assistants are Bupleurum which courses the qi and Corydalis which stops pain. Taken as a whole, this formula dispels cold and resolves congelation, quickens the blood and stops pain.

3. Clearing heat & transforming stasis method

When used together, medicinals for clearing heat and quickening the blood are indicated for burning heat and aching and pain in the chest, lateral costal regions, epigastrium, and abdomen with internal heat causing vexation and oppression, tension and agitation, easy anger, a purple tongue with yellow coating, and a wiry pulse. One commonly used formula is *Tao Hua Si Wu Tang* (Persica & Carthamus Four Materials Decoction) with added flavors, using a large amount of uncooked Radix Rehmanniae (*Sheng Di*) and adding Rhizoma Polygoni Cuspidati (*Hu Zhang*). If warm heat evils have invaded the constructive and blood, then the formula to use is *Xi Jiao Di Huang Tang* (Rhinoceros Horn & Rehmannia Decoction). If there is static heat in the lungs, then one should use *Qing Xuan Yu Re Tang* (Clear & Diffuse Static Heat Decoction). This method can be used for blood heat and septicemia, many types of circulatory diseases, lung abscess, bronchiectasis, hepatitis, and so forth.

Treatment principles: Clear heat and resolve toxins, quicken the blood and dispel stasis

Rx: Cornu Rhinocerotis (*Xi Jiao* for ecological reasons, [substitute Cornu Bubabli, *Shui Niu Jiao*]), 1g, Herba Lycopi Lucidi (*Ze Lan*), 9g, Herba Patriniae Heterophyllae (*Bai Jiang Cao*), 15g, Herba Lysimachiae Christinae (*Xian Ren Dui Zuo Cao*), 30g, Herba Ardisiae Japonicae (*Ping Di Mu*), 15g

Indications: Hepatitis B, septicemia, hemorrhagic disorders due to blood heat, circulatory diseases

Formula rationale: New diseases are in the channels; enduring diseases enter the network vessels. If liver depression has endured for many days, it will necessarily transform into fire. In that case, it is commonly seen in clinical practice that stasis and heat join and smolder. In this formula, Lycopus and Ardisia clear heat and quicken the blood. Rhinoceros Horn resolves toxins and opens the network vessels. This is assisted by Patrinia and Lysimachia which course the liver and quicken the blood, clear heat and disinhibit dampness. Taken as a whole, this formula clears heat and resolves toxins in the midst of quickening the blood.

4. Opening the network vessels & transforming stasis method

When used together, medicinals for opening the network vessels and medicinals which quicken the blood are appropriate for use when there is acute aching pain in the joints of the limbs whose bending and stretching is inhibited. This pain is mild in the day but severe at night. The commonly used formulas are *Huo Luo Xiao Ling Dan* (Miraculously Effective Open the Network Elixir) and *Shen Tong Zhu Yu Tang* (Body Pain Dispel Stasis Decoction). This method is indicated for the treatment of rheumatoid arthritis, hypertrophy of the cervical vertebrae, sciatica, and aching and pain of the joints of the four limbs caused by external injury.

Treatment principles: Quicken the blood and transform stasis, soften the hard and open the network vessels

Rx: Semen Strychnotis (*Ma Qian Zi*), 30g, Lumbricus (*Di Long*), 30 g, Cinnabar (*Zhu Sha*), 0.3 g, Eupolyphaga Seu Ophisthoplatia (*Di Bie Chong*), 3 g, Buthus Martensi (*Quan Xie*), 3 g

Indications: Rheumatoid arthritis, hypertrophy of the cervical vertebrae, periarthritis of the shoulder, lumbar muscle taxation and detriment

Formula rationale: Semen Strychnotis quickens the blood and opens the network vessels, disperses swelling and stops pain. It is the sovereign. Eupolyphaga breaks the blood and attacks stasis, disperses concretions and scatters nodulations. It is the minister. Earthworm dispels wind and resolves tremors. Scorpion opens the network vessels and scatters nodulation. These are the assistants. These are made into pills and coated with sugar. When these medicinals are used together, they have the power to quicken the blood and stop pain, dispel wind and open the network vessels.

5. Eliminating phlegm & quickening the blood method

When used together, medicinals for eliminating phlegm and medicinals for quickening the blood are indicated for the treatment of wind stroke paralysis, chest pain with cough and phlegm mixed with blood, chest *bi*, distention, and pain radiating to the upper back, a purple tongue with a slimy coating, and a wiry, slippery pulse. For wind stroke, *Zhi Mi Fu Ling Wan* (Fat Enchanting Poria Pills) and *Tao Hong Si Wu Tang* (Persica & Carthamus Four Materials Decoction) are used. For lung abscess, use *Quan Wei Jing Tang* (Whole Phragmites Decoction). For chest *bi*, use *Gua Lou Xie Bai Bai Jiu Tang* (Trichosanthes, Allium, & Alcohol Decoction) plus Hirudo (*Shui Zhi*). For transforming phlegm, the commonly used medicinals are uncooked Rhizoma Pinelliae Ternatae (*Ban Xia*), Retinervus Fascicularis Citri Reticulatae (*Ju Luo*), Semen Sinapis Albae (*Bai Jie Zi*), and Rhizoma Pleionis (*Shan Ci Gu*). For transforming stasis, the commonly used medicinals are Rhizoma Ligustici Wallichii (*Chuan Xiong*), Radix Rubrus Paeoniae Lactiflorae (*Chi Shao*), Semen Pruni Persicae (*Tao Ren*), and Flos Carthami Tinctorii (*Hong Hua*). This method is indicated for use in hypertension, coronary heart diseases, hyperlipidemia, senile bronchitis, cardiopulmonary disease, and epilepsy.

Treatment principles: Quicken the blood and dispel stasis, downbear the qi and transform phlegm

Rx: Herba Sargassii (*Hai Zao*), 9g, uncooked Pollen Typhae (*Pu Huang*), 9g, lime(-processed) Rhizoma Pinelliae Ternatae (*Fa Ban Xia*), Retinervus Fascicularis Citri Reticulatae (*Ju Luo*), 3g, Radix Ligustici Wallichii (*Chuan Xiong*), 9g, Radix Rubrus Paeoniae Lactiflorae (*Chi Shao*), 9g, Semen Pruni Persicae (*Tao Ren*), 9g, Flos Carthami Tinctorii (*Hong Hua*), 9g, Fructus Crataegi (*Shan Zha*), 9g, Fructus Perillae Frutescentis (*Su Zi*), 9g

Indications: Coronary heart disease, hypertension, wind stroke, senile dementia

Formula rationale: Fluids and blood have a common source, and blood stagnation leads to the formation of blood stasis. If fluids stop they will produce phlegm. Thus phlegm and stasis are mutually related. In this formula, Ligusticum, Pollen Typhae, Red Peony, Persica, and Carthamus quicken the blood and transform stasis. Sargassium, Orange Retinervus, and Pinellia dispel phlegm. These are combined with Crataegus which assists the power of quickening the blood at the same time as it harmonizes the stomach qi. These are also assisted by Perilla Seed in order to increase the power of transforming phlegm. It also downbears the qi.

6. Softening the hard & transforming stasis method

When used together, medicinals for softening the hard and medicinals that quicken the blood are indicated for the treatment of goiter and scrofula, phlegm nodulation, and concretions and conglomerations, accumulations and gatherings. Commonly used formulas are *Ren Shen Bie Jia Qian Wan* (Ginseng & Carapax Amydae Pills), *Xiao Lou Jiao Wan* (Disperse Scrofula Pills), *Da Huang Zhe Chong Wan* (Rhubarb & Eupolyphaga Pills), and *Gui Zhi Fu Ling Wan* (Cinnamon Twig & Poria Pills). For softening the hard and scattering nodulation, the commonly used medicinals are Rhizoma Dioscoreae Bulbiferae (*Huang Yao Zi*), Herba Sargassii (*Hai Zao*), Thallus Algae (*Kun Bu*), Squama Manitis Pentadactylis (*Chuan Shan Jia*), and Semen Vaccariae Segetalis (*Wang

Bu Liu Xing). This method is indicated for enlargement of the spleen and liver, vascular tumors, uterine fibroids, ovarian cysts, prostatic hypertrophy, chronic pelvic inflammation, and cystic appendix.

Treatment principles: Move the qi and quicken the blood, soften the hard and scatter nodulation

Rx: Hirudo (*Shui Zhi*), Concha Ostreae (*Mu Li*), Rhizoma Corydalis Yanhusuo (*Yan Hu Suo*). Use equal parts, grind into powder, and make into pills with water. Take 3g each time, 3 times per day.

Indications: Vascular tumors, hepatomegaly, splenomegaly, prostatic hypertrophy, hemiplegia

Formula rationale: In cases of nodulation, swelling, and lumps, there is ususally stasis, depression, and phlegm all binding with each other and not scattering. If the evils remain for a long time, they enter the network vessels. Therefore, the medicinals used are all attacking and checking. In the above formula, Hirudo is the sovereign. Its nature likes movement. It breaks the blood and dispels stasis. It is able to dispel concretions and conglomerations, accumulations and gatherings due to old static blood. It is combined with Corydalis which moves the qi and quickens the blood and Oyster Shell which transforms phlegm and softens the hard. Thus together, these medicinals have the power to move the qi and quicken the blood, soften the hard and scatter nodulation.

7. Attacking, precipitating & transforming stasis method

When used together, medicinals for attacking and precipitating and medicinals which quicken the blood are indicated in case of lower abdominal hardness, fullness, and aching and pain which refuses pressure with constipation. There may also be mania or women may have amenorrhea or a lochia which is not precipitated. Commonly used formulas are *Tao He Cheng Qi Tang* (Persica Order the Qi Decoction),

Di Dang Tang (Resistance Decoction), *Kong Xian Dan* (Control Drool Elixir), and *Da Huang Mu Dan Tang* (Rhubard & Moutan Decoction). This method is indicated in ectopic pregnancy, appendicitis, pancreatitis, cholelithiasis, and various acute abdominal patterns.

Treatment principles: Quicken the blood and dispel stasis, open the secreted and eliminate accumulations

Rx: Radix Et Rhizoma Rhei (*Da Huang*), 9g, add toward the end of decocting the other medicinals, Semen Pruni Persicae (*Tao Ren*), 9g, Rhizoma Curcumae Zedoariae (*E Zhu*), 9g, Rhizoma Polygoni Cuspidati (*Hu Zhang*), 30g, Fructus Immaturus Citri Seu Ponciri (*Zhi Shi*), 9g, Radix Saussureae Seu Vladimiriae (*Mu Xiang*), 9g, Mirabilitum (*Yuan Ming Fen*), 3g, dissolved after the other medicinals have been decocted, Radix Rubrus Paeoniae Lactiflorae (*Chi Shao*), 9g, Cortex Magnoliae Officinalis (*Chuan Po*), 9g, Fructus Crataegi (*Shan Zha*), 15g

Indications: Acute cholecystitis and cholelithiasis, acute pancreatitis, acute appendicitis, etc.

Formula rationale: The six bowels can function when they are open. If food becomes stopped up and stagnant within them, this will necessarily lead to qi and blood's transportation and movement suffering obstruction. Thus the qi becomes stagnant and the blood becomes static. Therefore, *Da Cheng Qi Tang* is designed to free the flow of the stools and eliminate accumulations. Persica, Zedoaria, Polygonum Cupidatum, and Red Peony quicken the blood and dispel stasis. They are assisted by Saussurea which moves the qi. Thus nodulations are scattered and stasis is transformed. These are aided by Crataegus which disperses food accumulations. When these medicinals are used together, they achieve a good effect in quickening the blood and dispelling stasis, opening the secreted and eliminating accumulations.

8. Stopping bleeding & transforming stasis method

When used together, stopping bleeding medicinals and quickening the blood medicinals are indicated for hemoptysis, hematemsis, and epistaxis when the color of the blood is purplish and black, if it is fresh red but contains lumps, or if there are bloody stools like lacquer. The commonly used medicinals are substances like Pollen Typhae (*Pu Huang*), Radix Et Rhizoma Rhei (*Da Huang*), Radix Pseudoginseng (*San Qi*), etc. This method is indicated for the treatment of upper digestive tract bleeding, various types of hemorrhaging, gynecological dribbling and mensturation which will not stop, and other hemorrhagic diseases.

Treatment principles: Clear heat and stop bleeding, transform stasis and quiet the network vessels

Rx: Uncooked Pollen Typhae (*Pu Huang*), Radix Rumicis (*Tu Da Huang*), Rhizoma Bletillae Striatae (*Bai Ji*). Equal amounts of these are ground into powder. Take 4.5g each time, 3 times per day.

Indications: Upper digestive tract bleeding and various types of hemorrhagic diseases

Formula rationale: Uncooked Pollen Typhae transforms stasis and stops bleeding. Rumex drains fire and stops bleeding. These are assisted by Bletilla which restrains spillage of the blood and stops bleeding. It also astringes long-standing sores. The use of these three medicinals together is based on empirical experience.

9. Boosting the qi & transforming stasis method

When used together, medicinals which supplement the qi and quicken the blood are indicated for the treatment of chest, lateral costal, epigastric, and abdominal insidious, lingering pain. If there is over-taxation, this pain is aggravated. There may also be hemiplegia, shortness of breath, lack of strength, a pale, purplish tongue, and a choppy, forceless pulse. Commonly used formulas are *Bu Yang Huan Wu Tang* (Supplement Yang & Restore the Five [Viscera] Decoction), *Huang Qi Si Wu Tang* (Astragalus Four Materials Decoction), and *Yi Xin Tang* (Boost the Heart Decoction: Radix Codonopsis Pilosulae [*Dang Shen*], Radix Astragali Membranacei [*Huang Qi*], Radix Ligustici Wallichii [*Chuan Xiong*], Radix Puerariae [*Ge Gen*], Fructus Crataegi [*Shan Zha*], Lignum Dalbergiae Odoriferae [*Jiang Xiang*], Radix Salviae Miltiorrhizae [*Dan Shen*], Rhizoma Acori Graminei [*Chang Pu*], stir-fried Semen Cassiae Torae [*Jue Ming Zi*]). This method is indicated for the treatment of chronic diseases which will not heal even with prolonged treatment, coronary heart disease, chronic hepatitis, cirrhosis of the liver, ulcerative diseases, the sequelae of wind stroke, and a variety of functional diseases.

Treatment principles: Boost the qi and transform stasis, quicken the blood and open the network vessels

Rx: Radix Astragali Membranacei (*Huang Qi*), 30g, Rhizoma Atractylis (*Cang Zhu*), 9g, Radix Ligustici Wallichii (*Chuan Xiong*), 9g, Flos Carthami Tinctorii (*Hong Hua*), 9g, Radix Rubrus Paeoniae Lactiflorae (*Chi Shao*), 9g, Semen Pruni Persicae (*Tao Ren*), 9g, Radix Angelicae Sinensis (*Dang Gui*), 9g, Radix Bupleuri (*Chai Hu*), 9g, uncooked Pollen Typhae (*Pu Huang*), 9g, wrapped during decoction

Indications: Coronary heart disease, chronic hepatitis, the sequelae of wind stroke

Formula rationale: If qi moves, the blood moves. If qi is vacuous, blood flow will not be uninhibited. Thus various diseases will be engendered. Astragalus is the ruler in this formula and it supplements the qi. It is assisted by Atractylodes which promotes transportation and transformation. This then results in the quickening of the blood and transformation of stasis, the supporting of the righteous and the out-thrusting of evils. "If qi is free-flowing and blood is quickened, there is nothing that cannot be eliminated." Balancing the qi and blood is especially effective in the treatment of chronic diseases of the elderly.

10. Fostering yin & transforming stasis method

When used together, medicinals for enriching and nourishing yin and medicinals which quicken the blood are indicated in cases with a dark, blackish, lusterless facial complexion, scaly, dry skin, vexatious heat in the five hearts, racing heart, scant sleep, insidious, burning pain in the chest, lateral costal regions, epigastrium, and abdomen, a purplish red tongue with a peeled coating, and a fine, rapid pulse. If the disease is located in the channels and network vessels, one should use *Si Miao Yong An Tang* (Four Wonders Quickly Quieting Decoction). If the disease is in the viscera and bowels, one should use *Da Bu Yin Wan* (Great Supplementing Yin Pills) combined with *Tao Hong Si Wu Tang* (Persica & Carthamus Four Materials Decoction) or *Yi Guan Jian* (One Link Decoction) and *Xia Yu Xue Tang* (Precipitate Static Blood Decoction). This method is indicated in cirrhosis of the liver, chronic leukemia, phlebitis, tuberculosis, diabetes mellitus, and other chronic cachectic diseases.

Treatment principles: Enrich and nourish yin fluids, quicken the blood and soften the hard, dispel stasis and open the network vessels

Rx: Uncooked Carapax Amydae Sinensis (*Bie Jia*), 15g, decocted first, Radix Salviae Miltiorrhizae (*Dan Shen*), 15g, Radix Ilicis Pubescentis (*Mao Dong Qing*), 15g, uncooked Pollen Typhae (*Pu Huang*), 9g, wrapped during decoction, Rhizoma Curcumae Zedoariae (*E Zhu*), 9g, Semen Pruni Persicae (*Tao Ren*), 9g, Radix Rubrus Paeoniae Lactiflorae (*Chi Shao*), 9g, Cortex Radicis Moutan (*Dan Pi*), 9g, Radix Scrophulariae Ningpoensis (*Yuan Shen*), 9g

Indications: Cirrhosis of the liver, chronic leukemia

Formula rationale: Fostering yin is the root and transforming stasis is the branch. In this formula, Scrophularia, Carapax Amydae, Salvia, and Red Peony protect and nourish constructive yin, while Moutan, Zedoaria, Persica, Pollen Typhae, and Ilex course and open the pathways of stasis. Thus yin is fostered at the same time as evil heat is restrained from harassing the constructive. Therefore, yin and yang, qi and blood are returned to balance and harmony.

6
Formulas for Combating Senility & Preserving Health Based on the Balancing Method

1. Heng Fa Yi Hao (Balancing Method #1)

Rx: Flos Carthami Tinctorii (*Hong Hua*), 9g, Semen Pruni Persicae (*Tao Ren*), 9g, Radix Ligustici Wallichii (*Chuan Xiong*), 6g, Radix Platycodi Grandiflori (*Jie Geng*), 4.5g, Fructus Citri Seu Ponciri (*Zhi Qiao*), 4.5g, Radix Achyranthis Bidentatae (*Niu Xi*), 4.5g

Indications: Neurasthenia, hysteria, emotional depression, menopausal syndrome. This formula also can be used to help prevent senility.

Method of administration: The above ingredients are decocted and condensed down to 100ml of liquid. Fifty milliliters should be taken each time, 2 times per day.

Clinical results: Eighty cases manifested such different symptoms as insomnia, nightmare, poor memory, baldness, fatigue, dizziness, vexation and agitation, and tidal fever (*i.e.*, hot flashes). In these cases, sedatives had not been markedly effective. Therefore, the patients were given the above treatment. Based on their subjective symptoms, physical signs, and indices of blood rheology, the effects of this treatment were judged and classified as either markedly effective, fairly improved, or no result. In 46 cases, the therapeutic effect was pronounced. Their physical signs and symptoms disappeared, and their indices of blood rheology returned to normal. Thirty-four cases showed fair improvement. Their signs and symptoms were not improved, but their indices of blood rheology changed for the better. In one case, there was no effect at all. Blood rheology tests had a P value of less than 0.01. The process of improvement usually developed in sequence, with first the disappearance of symptoms, then the recovery of physical signs, and finally the return of normal indices of blood rheology.

Formula rationale: *Heng Fa Yi Hao* is based on indications suggested for Wang Qing-ren's Qing Dynasty *Xue Fu Zhu Yu Tang* (Blood Mansion Dispel Stasis Decoction) found in his *Yi Lin Gai Cuo (Corrections of Mistakes in the Medical Forest)*. Presented with the indications for that formula, Master Wang said, "All prior formulas are not responsive", "The hundreds of formulas are ineffectual", and "In treatment, none of them is effective." Based on my several decades of clinical experience, I believe that the lack of results in most such cases is because the physician has simply treated neurasthenia by calming the nerves and has neglected such disease causes as the patient's mental/emotional lack of relaxation and liver qi depression and stagnation.

TCM holds that the heart treasures the spirit, while the liver stores the ethereal soul. If the heart is diseased, the spirit cannot depend on it. If there is liver depression, the ethereal soul cannot rely on that organ. Their vow is not fulfilled. Qi and blood become congealed and obstructed. The brain qi and the visceral qi do not connect. Spirit and ethereal soul are not retained. It is thus necessary to treat this disease by disinhibiting and opening the channels and network vessels, regulating and harmonizing the viscera and bowels, and balancing qi and blood so that the functions of the five internal viscera will return to their proper places.

After administering *Heng Fa Yi Hao*, subjective symptoms, physical signs, and the results of modern laboratory tests all change for the better. Therefore, this therapy is consistent with the aim of nourishing life in the *Nei Jing (Inner Classic)*. In other words, form and spirit are both treated.

In this formula, Carthamus, Persica, and Ligusticum form the nucleus for transforming stasis. Platycodon is used to carry the other medicinals and move them upward. Citrus smooths and disinhibits the middle region, and Achyranthes conducts the medicinals and moves them downward. Thus qi and blood may pass and flow freely from the upper, through the middle, and to the lower region, and there is no fear that stasis may remain behind. Because the qi flows freely and the blood is quickened, the functions of the five viscera are able to be regulated. Thus, owing to stability in the internal environment, various symptoms manifesting in the nervous system can be automatically cured without receiving specific treatment.

In my experience, functional diseases of the nervous system belong to the category of internal damage by the emotions and orientation. Such pathological changes are closely related to the heart and liver. At first, the disease is mostly replete. It is characterized mainly by the symptoms of the six depressions. In particular, qi and blood depression and stagnation are the pivotal point in such disease. If the disease endures, it will change from repletion to vacuity. Clinically, it is common to see vacuity and repletion at the same time, while yin and yang are perverse and disobedient.

The balancing method balances the qi and blood. Therefore, the symptoms may relax and resolve (*i.e.*, remit). This formula is able to treat extensively diseases in different systems and it does so based on the most fundamental premises regarding the treatment of disease in TCM. The formula *Heng Fa Yi Hao* has been used to treat many cases of obstinate insomnia. In these cases, sedatives have been ineffective, but administering this formula has produced marked effect. One patient reflected that, after taking this formula, he felt as if he were drunk. Later he fell asleep and felt very comfortable. In the day, he was not fatigued.

Clinically, this formula may also be used to treat and prevent schizo-phrenia. In this case, 30g of uncooked Iron (*Tie Luo*) or 9g of *Ci Zhu Wan* (Magnetite & Cinnabar Pills), wrapped during decoction, should be added to the decoction. In preventing schizophrenia, this decoction should be administered every other day. Based on several cases, the effects of this treatment prove satisfactory. In treating obstinate headache, the dose of Ligusticum in this formula recipe should be increased to 15g or even to more than 30g. This treatment has effective in many cases.

2. *Heng Fa Er Hao* (Balancing Method #2)

Rx: *Heng Fa Yi Hao* plus Radix Scutellariae Baicalensis (*Huang Qin*)

Indications: Common geriatric diseases such as arteriosclerosis, hypertension, hyperlipidemia, the sequelae of wind stroke, insufficient blood supply to the cerebral vessels, hypo-proteinemia, chronic bronchitis, prostatic hypertrophy, diseases of the cervical vertebrae, and premature senility

Method of administration: Same as for *Heng Fa Yi Hao*

Clinical results: A comparison was made before and after administration of this formula in 150 elderly patients. It showed that, in regards to the clinical symptoms of common geriatric diseases such as chest oppression, heart palpitations, insomnia, chest pain, cough, shortness of breath, dizziness, superficial edema in the lower limbs, devitalized appetite, essence spirit atony and torpor, and poor complexion, oral administration of 1 course of the formula *Heng Fa Er Hao* was able to markedly improve the above-mentioned clinical symptoms. Statistical analysis of data shows a P value of less than 0.01. Analysis by modern laboratory equipment of the morphology of nail bed microcirculation, capillary rheology, and the character of blood rheology show that this formula can markedly improve blood rheology, reduce the viscosity of the plasma, change capillary rheology, accelerate blood circulation, increase the beneficial blood supply to the viscera, help maintain normal physiological function, raise the immunity of the organism, promote the conversion rate of lymphocytes, strengthen resistance to disease, promote the anabolism of protein in the organism, raise protein in the serum, effectively maintain normal reproductive function, promote the discharge of metabolic wastes, and finally, to reduce pigmentation. Improvement in these physiological, biochemical, histological, immunological, and clinical indices of senility are all the results of coursing and disinhibiting as well as balancing the organism's qi and blood.

Formula rationale: In recent years, in order to explore the secrets of human senility and seek effective medicinals to delay it, many scholars at home and abroad have approached this problem from different angles and put forward various viewpoints. However, in the last analysis, none of these are different from the traditional theory on "vacuity detriment of the viscera and bowels." Through observation and research, the writer has confirmed that the chief causes of human senility are loss of regulation of the qi and blood, obstruction of the coursing and free flow of the channels and vessels, and static blood stopping and stagnating. Thus the balance of qi and blood is impaired by the presence of static blood. The viscera and bowels are not able to obtain their normal moistening and nourishment and hence various pathological changes associated with senility result.

It is then that there appear vacuity and debility in the viscera and bowels, essence, qi, and spirit deficiency and consumption, and diminishment of the qi's engendering and transforming function. This aggravates the formation of blood stasis and produces a vicious cycle which leads to senility and finally to death. Vacuity is but the branch, while stasis is the root. Therefore, in order to delay the senility of organism and maintain normal physiological function, one should resolve and eliminate the manifestations of static blood in the various viscera and bowels, thus enabling them to obtain their normal moisture and nourishment.

Heng Fa Er Hao is a formula derived from *Heng Fa Yi Hao*. In order to explore the anti-senility mechanism of *Heng Fa Er Hao*, I led a scientific research group in conducting animal experiments and established a control group for observation. The results of this research demonstrate that, through microscopic examination, the structure of the blood vessels and tissues in the anatomized viscera of the elderly rabbits given this formula was essentially the same as that of young rabbits. While in the control group, the condition was entirely different. In that group there were pathological changes such as marked trouble in capillary circulation, thickening of the vascular walls, constriction of the lumena, sedimentation of metabolic waste, and intercellular ecchymotic blood. This further explains that, through their coordinated function, the medicinals which boost the qi, quicken the blood, and transform stasis can not only rectify the signs of loss of balance of yin and yang but also produce incontrovertible effects on the senility of the organism.

In my experience, combating senility is nowadays an up-to-date, sophisticated subject in the field of medical biology. Undoubtedly, early senility adversely affects the length of life, while for people whose senility comes late, the possibility of longevity is of course great. Authoritative scientists around the world divide senility-combating methods into "primary prophylaxis" and "secondary prophylaxis." This classification is essentially the same as that expressed in the *Nei Jing (Inner Classic)*, namely, "to prevent diseases before they occur" and "to prevent their secondary changes (when they have already occurred)." *Heng Fa Er Hao* is formulated on precisely this basis. Qi vacuity and blood stasis are the root of the pathological changes this formula addresses.

If qi depression transforms into fire, then it should be combined with Cortex Radicis Moutan (*Dan Pi*) and Fructus Gardeniae Jasminoidis (*Shan Zhi*) to clear the liver and discharge fire. If qi depression is accompanied by phlegm, then it should be combined with Pericarpium Viridis Citri Reticulatae (*Qing Pi*) and Fructus Trichosanthis Kirlowii (*Gua Lou*) to transform phlegm and scatter nodulation. If there is both blood stasis and dampness, it should be combined with Rhizoma Atractylodis Macrocephalae (*Bai Zhu*) and Rhizoma Alismatis (*Ze Xie*) in order to fortify the transportation and disinhibition of dampness. If blood stasis is accompanied by food accumulation, then it should be combined with Rhizoma Curcumae Zedoariae (*E Zhu*) and Rhizoma

Sparganii (*San Leng*) in order to grind accumulation and disperse food. In addition, depending upon the disease conditions, Semen Ziziphi Spinosae (*Suan Zao Ren*) can be used to boost one's intelligence, nourish the heart, and quiet the spirit. Rhizoma Atractylodis Macrocephalae (*Bai Zhu*) and Sclerotium Poriae Cocos (*Fu Ling*) may be added to supplement the qi and fortify the spleen. And Rhizoma Curculiginis Orchoidis (*Xian Mao*) and Herba Epimedii (*Xian Ling Pi*) may be added to supplement and boost the *chong* and *ren*.

3. *Heng Fa San Hao* (Balancing Method #3)

Rx: Radix Astragali Membranacei (*Huang Qi*), 30g Radix Codonopsis Pilosulae (*Dang Shen*), 15g, Radix Scutellariae Baicalensis (*Huang Qin*), 15g, Radix Puerariae (*Ge Gen*), 9g, Radix Rubrus Paeoniae Lactiflorae (*Chi Shao*), 9g, Radix Ligustici Wallichii (*Chaun Xiong*), 9g, Radix Salviae Miltiorrhizae (*Dan Shen*), 15g, Fructus Crataegi (*Shan Zha*), 30g, Seman Cassiae Torae (*Jue Ming Zi*), 30g.

Indications: Coronary heart diseases, heart arrhythmia, occlusive cerebral vascular disease. Can also be used to delay senility.

Method of administration: Same as for *Heng Fa Yi Hao*

Clinical results: Forty-eight cases with coronary heart disease were selected as subjects for study with this formula. Before administration of the formula, electrocardiogram (EKG) showed abnormal phenomena in 35 cases or 72%. Among these, there are 20 cases of change in ST-T segment, 7 cases of paroxysmal auricular premature beat, 5 cases of paroxysmal ventricular premature beat, and 3 cases of auricular fibrillation. After a course of treatment with the above formula, EKG still showed abnormal phenomena in 5 cases. In 3 cases the ST-T segment remained unchanged. There was 1 case of auricular fibrillation and 1 case of paroxysmal ventricular premature beat, accounting for 10.4%. By statistical analysis, the P value was less than 0.01. This study, therefore, showed a very marked significance. Another study of

51 cases with irregular cardiac rhythm showed that, simultaneous with improvement of symptoms after a course of treatment with this formula, the concentration of blood platelets was also markedly reduced. This may be the reason why this formula can produce effects not only on bradycardia but also on tachycardia. Through observation, this formula has also proven effective in most cases with occlusive cerebral vascular disease.

Formula rationale: In the TCM medicinal treatment of coronary heart disease, irregular cardiac rhythm, and occlusive cerebral vascular disease, most scholars in our country nowadays use the methods of quickening the blood and transforming stasis, diffusing *bi* and opening yang, and breaking up phlegm and scattering nodulations. It is my opinion that, in terms of these diseases' causes and mechanisms, vacuity is the root and repletion is the branch. Based on heart qi vacuity being the root and static blood being the branch, I believe that one should mainly use boosting the qi, quickening the blood, and transforming stasis treatment.

Clinical surveys have shown that the above formula quickly ameliorates the symptoms of coronary heart disease, angina pectoris, and cerebral arteriosclerosis. Electrocardiography demonstrates that the rate of return to normal with this formula is high. When a person becomes old, their qi and blood are insufficient and their viscera and bowels lose their nourishment. Therefore, the signs of visceral vacuity and debility as well as internal stoppage of static blood appear. The disease mechanism in most cases is heart qi insufficiency and phlegm stasis joining and obstructing the vessels and network vessels.

This formula uses large amounts of Codonopsis and Astragalus as its sovereigns to nourish the heart and boost the qi. These are accompanied by Pueraria, Ligusticum, Salvia, Red Peony, and Crataegus as the ministers to quicken the blood and open the vessels. These sovereigns and ministers act in concert to boost the qi and quicken the blood so that, when qi is sufficient, it will help the blood to move and when it moves, static blood is eliminated. Cassia acts as the assistant in coursing and opening, ascending and descending the qi mechanism, thus increasing the power of quickening the blood. Therefore, this formula simultaneously supplements and frees the flow. As Shen Jin-ao said, "Supplementing, boosting, and attacking, alternating and occurring simultaneously, this is the right way to treat disease."

In my experience, if stasis obstructs the heart vessels and there is acute chest pain, then equal amounts of powdered Radix Pseudoginseng (*San Qi*) and Sanguis Draconis (*Xue Jie*) should be mixed together and stirred evenly. One may administer 1.5g of this each time or 9g of *Shi Xiao San* (Sudden Smile Powder). Four point five grams of Resina Olibani (*Ru Xiang*) and the same weight of Resina Myrrhae (*Mo Yao*) should also be administered. If pain still is not ameliorated, 0.03g of Secretio Moschi Moschiferi (*She Xiang*), washed down by the other medicinals, should be added to open the channels, quicken the blood, and stop pain. If there is chest oppression, 4.5g of Fructus Citri Seu Ponciri (*Zhi Qiao*) and the same weight of Radix Achyranthis Bidentatae (*Niu Xi*) should be used, one to upbear and one to downbear, thus regulating and disinhibiting the qi mechanism and freeing the flow of chest yang. If there is phlegm congestion and qi stagnation with chest *bi* pain which spreads to the upper back, then 15g of Fructus Trichosanthis Kirlowii (*Gua Lou*) and 9g of Bulbus Allii Macrostemi (*Xie Bai*) should be used to diffuse *bi* and open binding. If there is qi vacuity and yang detriment with greenish blue face and purple lips, perspiration, and chilled limbs, add Radix Panacis Ginseng (*Ren Shen*), 9g, and Radix Lateralis Praeparatus Aconiti Carmichaeli (*Fu Zi*), 6g, to warm yang and open the vessels. If qi and yin are both damaged and the mouth is dry and the tongue coating is scant, then Tuber Ophiopogonis Japonicae (*Mai Dong*), 9g, Rhizoma Polygonati Odorati (*Yu Zhu*), 12g, and Fructus Schisandrae Chinensis (*Wu Wei Zi*), 4.5g, should be added or one should combine this formula with *Sheng Mai San* (Engender the Pulse Powder) and *Tian Wang Bu Xin Dan* (Heavenly Emperor Supplement the Heart Elixir) in order to boost the qi and nourish yin, restore the pulse and quiet the spirit.

4. *Heng Fa Si Hao* (Balancing Method #4)

Rx: *Heng Fa Yi Hao* plus Fluoritum (*Zi Shi Ying*), 30g, Semen Allii Tuberosi (*Jiu Cai Zi*), 9g, prepared Radix Rehmanniae (*Shu Di*), 12g

Indications: Manifestations of early senility, such as early decline in the male's sexual function, atrophy of the genitalia and the tissue of the female's breasts

Method of administration: The same as for *Heng Fa Yi Hao*

Clinical results: This formula achieves relatively good results in maintaining the reproductive function of the organism. In animal experiments treating male rabbits with the formula *Heng Fa Si Hao* for 2 ½ years, there was no evidence under microscopic examination of any atrophy of their seminal tubules nor any marked degeneration of spermatocytes at any of various stages. The structure of these cells and their nuclei were quite distinct, and the spermatozoa were rather numerous. In the control group, there was marked degeneration. In the group administered this formula, the uteri of the female rabbits were still hypertrophic, while their endometria were thickened. AKP chromosomes were negative. These rabbits, aged 2 ½ years, still retained their normal sexual behavior and sexual function. In the control group, degeneration in this behavior and function was pronounced.

Clinical practice also confirms that the formula *Heng Fa Si Hao* does produce certain definite effects on premature senility of the genitals and sexual dysfunction, including male impotence, premature ejaculation, inability to ejaculate, and atrophy of the scrotum as well as female loss of sexual desire and flabbiness of the breasts. This method has been used to treat two such cases. In one case, the patient did not ejaculate semen for 11 years. In the other, their scrotum had atrophied. The attending physician referred to this as a "strange disease (*guai bing*)." Both TCM and Western drugs had been extensively applied but without any effect. We then administered more than 20 packets of this formula and finally achieved success.

Formula rationale: In my clinical practice, I have employed quickening the blood and transforming stasis to regulate loss of balance of the organism in the treatment of geriatric diseases which are traditionally considered due to kidney vacuity as well as being a manifestation of premature senility in the reproductive and sexual functions. The kidneys treasure the essence and govern the marrow, while the brain is the sea of marrow and governs the higher central nervous activities.

However, treating the brain is tantamount to treating the heart. The heart governs the vessels and the vessels are the mansion of the blood. In this formula, Citrus courses and rectifies the qi mechanism. *Tao Hong Si Wu Tang* (Persica & Carthamus Four Materials Decoction) quickens the blood and transforms stasis. Platycodon and Achyranthes disinhibit above and below and pass through and open the blood vessels. Fluoritum stimulates the yang pathways. Prepared Rehmannia fills the essence and boosts the marrow. Therefore, after treatment with this formula, the essence spirit of patients with the above-mentioned diseases is markedly improved.

This regulation of cerebral excitation and inhibition itself conduces to the establishment of the conditioned reflexes which are the normal activities of sexual function. The *Nei Jing (Inner Classic)* says, "If the qi vessels are always free-flowing, the kidney qi will have a surplus." Yang obtains yin and there is engenderment. Yin obtains yang and there is free flow. When yin and yang combine their virtues, they execute their transformation and production. In the treatment of male sexual troubles and female frigidity, one frequently sees the use of Radix Panacis Ginseng (*Ren Shen*), Cornu Parvum Cervi (*Lu Rong*), and gonadotrophin. In fact, if stasis and stagnation join and bind, qi loses its coursing and inhibition, and the kidneys lose their nourishment. If the disease endures for many days, not only will the symptoms not improve, but one's personality and behavior will also become eccentric. This is a great misfortune.

In my experience, current medical theory already supports the view that troubles in male sexual function are due to loss of regulation and spreading in the qi mechanism and loss of coursing and disinhibition in the blood vessels. For instance, senile impotence is often a secondary disease of the branching main artery and atherosclerosis of the large vessels in the pelvis.

Additions & subtractions to this formula: For impotence, add Fructus Cnidii Monnieri (*She Chuang Zi*). For premature ejaculation, remove the Achyranthes and Fluoritum and add Cortex Phellodendri (*Huang Bai*) and Rhizoma Anemarrhenae (*Zhi Mu*). For failure to ejaculate, Squama Manitis Pentadactylis (*Chuan Shan Jia*) and Semen Vaccariae Segetalis (*Wang Bu Liu Xing*) should be added. For atrophy of convoluted seminal cells, add Rhizoma Curculiginis Orchioidis (*Xian Mao*) and Herba Epimedii (*Xian Ling Pi*), 9g. each.

7
Secret Essentials in the Treatment of Commonly Seen Geriatric Patterns

Senility is an inevitable physiological process due to the aging of tissues and cells and the decline in organ function which accompany advancing years. The aim of nourishing life is to enable one to live out their heaven(-decreed) years and avoid premature death. It is a fact that senility markedly raises the incidence of disease in the elderly. Therefore, the treatment of disease in the elderly is an important method for promoting one's longevity. In seeking the best method of treatment in the aged, if one only uses "patterns" according to the theory of TCM or "diseases" based on modern Western medicine, regarding these as their general outline for classification, then each system of categorization has its strong and weak points. From the macroscopic or intuitive point of view, in terms of the commonly seen patterns in the elderly, vacuity is the chief, and geriatric diseases lead to obvious functional impediment. However, from the microscopic point of view, pattern discrimination reveals repletion. Thus, in order to accurately reflect the true features of both diseases and patterns, it is necessary to keep in mind the idea that "patterns and diseases mutually supplement each other." Therefore, by juxtaposing diseases with patterns, and in addition, by taking into account disease causes and disease mechanisms, one should seek a unity between these two (*i.e.*, patterns and diseases).

Because, the conditions for the onset of disease and pathological changes in the human body are very complicated and, in addition, the mechanisms for senility have not yet all been fully elucidated, therefore, it seems difficult to discuss "diseases" together with "patterns." However, that does not mean there is no way to solve this difficulty. Starting from the premise that loss of balance of the qi and blood is the basis for pathological change, we can not only unravel the mystery of senility but also reveal the cause of diseases. Therefore, we can say that regulating and disciplining the balance of the qi and blood is the "essential" means to prevent and treat disease and to restore health. This is exactly my purpose in elaborating and demonstrating the methods of quickening the blood and transforming stasis. And herein lies the "secret."

From clinical experience, it is apparent that the elderly commonly feel deficient and vacuous after becoming diseased. Because pattern discrimination and the use of medicinals which that leads to is lacking, since traditional formulas for combating senility unduly emphasize enriching, supplementing, and strengthening, and since various types of symptoms have been neglected in pathological conditions, thus various harmful effects have been produced. These have often caused the existing low level of imbalance in the organism to become even more lop-sided, changing mild diseases into serious ones and serious diseases into death. As Xu Ling-tai, the famous Qing Dynasty doctor, has pointed out in the *Sheng Ji Chu Yan (The Sayings of a Cautious Doctor)*, "Since the qi and blood of the elderly do not flow very uninhibitedly, how can they bear supplementation which keeps the evils, thus making difficulties with the qi and blood?"

The substance of senility consists of blood stasis. Blood stasis is the foundation of the pathophysiology of geriatric diseases. Thus we have consistently based our approach on improving the capillary circulation of the organism, clearing and eliminating the phenomenon of blood stasis from the organism, restoring the internal environment to balance, and, in the end, effectively preventing and treating disease.

In preventing and treating geriatric diseases, we should first find our basis in the literature. As "The Treatise on the Secret Law of the Spiritual Orchid" in the *Su Wen (Simple Questions)* says, "Blockage and obstruction of the pathways and lack of free flow greatly damage the form." "The Treatise on Heat Disease" in the *Su Wen (Simple Questions)* further says, "If the three yin and three yang and the five viscera and six bowels all suffer disease, constructive and defensive will not move, the five viscera will not be free flowing, and thus death will occur." Whether due to external invasion or internal damage, blood stasis is the direct cause of disease and even death.

Through clinical practice, our knowledge and understanding has been gradually deepened. The diseases which we first selected included coronary angina pectoris, pulmonary heart disease, cirrhosis of the liver, and apoplexy due to lack of blood. The symptoms of blood stasis are all pronounced in these diseases, and our therapeutic results were satisfactory. Later, we extended the application of our method to long-standing and strange diseases, such as the slow resolution of pneumonia, senile psychosis, and scleroderma.

In addition, we have discovered the specific effects of medicinals which quicken the blood and transform stasis. This specificity has been observed through examining improvement in blood constituents and in the character and condition of the blood vessels. With the deepening of our scientific research, from physiology to pathology to pharmacology, we have not only proved the therapeutic efficacy of medicinals for quickening the blood and transforming stasis in the case of common geriatric diseases, but we have also eliminated from our minds the mystery of these medicinals. This mechanism has been described above and does not bear repeating here.

Up to now, our conclusion is as follows: I believe that in treating geriatric diseases characterized by marked symptoms of static blood, one should primarily use the methods of quickening the blood and transforming stasis. Whereas, in geriatric diseases which do not present obvious symptoms of static blood or in which symptoms of static blood are not pronounced, one should mainly rely on treatment given on the basis of pattern discrimination combined with medicinals which quicken the blood and transform stasis. It is my experience that this latter method can improve therapeutic results in geriatric diseases even without marked symptoms of static blood. In other words, no matter whether the disease is due to internal damage or external invasion, one can achieve better therapeutic results in the elderly if one routinely adds medicinals which quicken the blood and transform stasis to formulas otherwise correctly chosen based on TCM pattern discrimination alone. This is the secret essence of my method of treating geriatric disease.

1. Common cold (*Gan Mao*)

The term *gan mao* or common cold appears in the "Chapter on Various Winds" in the *Ren Zhao Zhi Zhi Fang (Direct Formulas from the Study of Mercy)*: "*Gan mao* wind evils: fever, headache, loud cough, pasty, sticky nasal mucous." This disease may occur all year round. Owing to changes of qi in the four seasons, disease evils and their symptoms are not all the same. When combined with the body's strength or weakness, treatment should be administered according to the mildness or severity of the invading evils. External evils may be mild or superficial, wind damage having stopped its invasion in the skin and hair. This is called common cold. However, if the patient is affected by unseasonable evil qi, this is known as epidemic influenza. At first, there mostly appears headache, nasal congestion, runny nose, sneezing, and fear of cold. Later, there will be fever and sore throat or cough and itchy throat. If serious, the fever will be high, the patient may detest cold, and their entire body may be sore and painful. In treating this disease, one should first discriminate wind cold from wind heat. Then one should mainly course wind, diffuse the lungs, and resolve the exterior. This should be aided by quickening the blood medicinals to achieve an even better effect.

Disease causes, disease mechanisms

This pathocondition often occurs when the weather suddenly changes or when cold and warmth lose their normalcy. If one lives imprudently and neglects such changes in cold and heat, if they become wet through in the rain or worn out with fatigue, then the body's interstices may become relaxed and their defensive qi then fails to secure. In that case, wind evils may take advantage of vacuity and invade the body. Because the elderlys' resistance to diseases is weak, after catching cold, the patient may present different complicated symptom complexes. As the proverb says, "The aged fear damage by cold (*i.e.*, external afflictions), while the young are afraid of consumptive disease." According to TCM, in different seasons, wind evils commonly combine with the seasonal qi when they invade the body. For instance, in winter, wind evils are mostly categorized as wind cold. In spring, wind evils are categorized as wind heat. In damp seasons, they mostly come along with dampness. In summer, they mostly come along with summerheat. In autumn, they mostly come along with dryness. Generally, however, this patho-condition may be divided into the two great patterns of wind cold and wind heat. Patterns accompanied with dampness, summerheat, and dryness are categorized as simultaneous (*i.e.*, mixed) patterns.

Treatment based on pattern discrimination

A. Wind cold

Main symptoms: Stuffy nose, bodily heaviness, sneezing, runny nose, cough with itchy throat, excessive, watery, thin phlegm, if severe, aversion to cold, fever, headache, generalized pain, no perspiration, a thin, white tongue coating, and a floating or floating, tight pulse

Treatment principles: Use acrid and warm ingredients to resolve the exterior, diffuse the lungs, and quicken the blood

Rx: Herba Schizonepetae Tenuifoliae (*Jing Jie*), 9g, Radix Lede-bouriellae Sesloidis (*Fang Feng*), 9g, uncooked Rhizoma Zingiberis (*Sheng Jiang*), 2 slices, Radix Ligustici Wallichii (*Chuan Xiong*), 4.5g, Radix Peucedani (*Qian Hu*), 9g, Radix Bupleuri (*Chai Hu*), 4.5g, Radix Platycodi Grandiflori (*Jie Geng*), 4.5g, Fructus Citri Seu Ponciri (*Zhi*

Qiao), 4.5g, Sclerotium Poriae Cocos (*Fu Ling*), 9g, Radix Et Rhizoma Notopterygii (*Qiang Huo*), 9g, Radix Salviae Miltiorrhizae (*Dan Shen*), 9g

B. Wind heat

Main symptoms: Fever, slight aversion to wind and cold, perspiration, generalized fever may not be obvious, headache, stuffy nose with turbid discharge, dry mouth and thirst, red, swollen, aching and painful throat, cough with yellow phlegm, a thin, yellow tongue coating, and a floating, rapid pulse

Treatment principles: Use acrid, cool medicinals to resolve the exterior, diffuse the lungs, and quicken the blood

Rx: Folium Mori Albi (*Sang Ye*), 9g, Flos Chrysanthemi Morifolii (*Ju Hua*), 9g, Radix Peucedani (*Qian Hu*), 9g, Semen Pruni Armeniacae (*Xing Ren*), 9g, Flos Lonicerae Japonicae (*Yin Hua*), 9g, Fructus Forsythiae Suspensae (*Lian Qiao*), 9g, Semen Praeparatum Sojae (*Dan Dou Chi*), 9g, Radix Rubrus Paeoniae Lactiflorae (*Chi Shao*), 9g, Radix Scutellariae Baicalensis (*Huang Qin*), 9g, Radix Isatidis Seu Baphicacanthi (*Ban Lan Gen*), 9g, Radix Salviae Miltiorrhizae (*Dan Shen*), 9g.

Secret essentials

1. In treating common cold in the aged, it is not appropriate to unduly emit and scatter. If the disease is lingering and cannot be cured, this is due to righteous qi vacuity and debility. It is, therefore, proper to add to the above formulas 9g of *Bu Zhong Yi Qi Wan* (Supplement the Center & Boost the Qi Pills), wrapped during decoction. If the disease relapses repeatedly, then one can regularly administer *Yu Ping Feng San* (Jade Wind Screen Powder), 6g each time, 2 times per day, in order to supplement the qi and boost the defensive. The effect is quite good.

2. Ready-made (or so-called patent) medicines for the common cold are generally acrid and cool and resolve the exterior. Their prolonged administration in the elderly is not appropriate. I typically use *Jia Wei Bu Zhong Yi Qi Tang* (Added Flavors Supplement the Center & Boost the Qi Decoction) from the *Bian Zheng Lu (Discriminating Patterns Record)*: Radix Astragali Membranacei (*Huang Qi*), 15g, Tuber Ophiopogonis Japonicae (*Mai Dong*), 9g, Rhizoma Atractylodis Macrocephalae (*Bai Zhu*), 9g, Radix Angelicae Sinensis (*Dang Gui*), 9g, Radix Codonopsis Pilosulae (*Dang Shen*), 9g, Radix Bupleuri (*Chai Hu*), 6g, Radix Trichosanthis Kirlowii (*Hua Fen*), 9g, Pericarpium Citri Reticulatae (*Chen Pi*), 6g, Sclerotium Poriae Cocos (*Fu Ling*), 9g, and Rhizoma Cimicifugae (*Sheng Ma*), 3g. This mainly treats common cold which will not heal in a vacuous person, easy catching of common cold which sometimes occur and sometimes cease. This formula follows the rule, "Support the righteous qi and evils will spontaneously be dispelled."

This formula's rationale is based on Astragalus boosting the qi and securing the exterior. Codonopsis, Atractylodes, and Radix Glycyrrhizae (*Gan Cao*) supplement the middle burner and fortify the spleen. Dang Gui nourishes and supplements the blood. Orange Peel rectifies the qi and transforms dampness. Cimicifuga raises and lifts yang qi. Poria transports the spleen and transforms turbidity. Dampness usually stagnates in a person who is internally vacuous. If a person's middle is vacuous there mostly is simultaneous stoppage of dampness. If dampness stagnates, spleen transportation will not be fortified and middle qi will become even weaker. If Trichosanthes and Ophiopogon are added to the formula, they will nourish lung yin and recede the fever. Then the effect of this formula will reach every aspect of this pattern's symptoms. Thus it is advisable to use this formula.

3. Because old peoples' bodies are weak, after catching a cold, its symptoms are not easily made manifest. When they have fever, it may not be obvious. When they catch cold, they may not appear markedly

abnormal. However, common cold is by no means a minor disease. It can lead to a recurrence of whatever chronic disease one may have. Therefore, one should not neglect it. A folk recipe is *Cong Jiang Zhou* (Scallion & Ginger Porridge). The ingredients consist of Herba Allii Fistulosi (*Cong Bai*), 3 stalks, uncooked Rhizoma Zingiberis (*Sheng Jiang*), 2 slices, Fructus Zizyphi Jujubae (*Hong Zao*), 10 pieces, and a handful of Semen Oryzae Sativae (*Geng Mi, i.e.,* polished rice). These are boiled together into porridge. The patient should eat 1 bowl of porridge each time to dispel the evil without damaging the righteous. At the beginning of the disease, if one uses this recipe, the disease will be eliminated as soon as the patient perspires. This prescription is not only economical but also convenient. Moreover, one avoids using medicinals of lop-sided nature and thus any harm such medicinals might cause.

2. Phlegm rheum (*Tan Yin*)

This disease often occurs in the elderly. Its chief symptoms are cough and panting (*i.e.* asthma). The phlegm is mostly white and frothy, hence the name "phlegm rheum." When phlegm rheum occurs, it usually endures and does not last for only a short period of time. It is caused by original qi vacuity with yin exuberance and yang debility. Thus fluids and humors congeal and stagnate and are not able to be transported and spread. These are retained and gather in the chest and middle. When water gathers, it becomes rheum. When rheum evils congeal, they become phlegm. Thus it is said, "Phlegm is produced from sticky, pasty rheum, while rheum is clear, watery phlegm." In fact, these two substances come from the same source. If the true origin is full and sufficient, the stomach is strong and the spleen is fortified. Therefore, drinking and eating will not lose their limits, and transportation and movement will not stop in the mechanism. How then can phlegm rheum be produced? Zhang Zhong-jing said, "For those diseased with phlegm rheum, warm medicinals should be used to harmonize." It is not appropriate only to break the qi or supplement with enriching, slimy medicinals. One should also not recklessly throw in sweet or cold medicinals which may greatly damage the spleen and stomach.

Disease causes, disease mechanisms

In the case of phlegm rheum cough, the disease resides in the lung channel. The lungs are the delicate viscus. They are responsible for clearing and depurating. If phlegm rheum radiates to the lungs, upward counterflow results in cough. The cause of phlegm rheum is the spleen and stomach's transportation and movement not reaching. Thus it is said, "The spleen is the source of phlegm engenderment, but the lungs are the reservoir of phlegm." Phlegm rheum cough in the elderly usually occurs in autumn when the weather suddenly becomes cool. The symptoms are usually aggravated with the severe cold of winter and gradually subside when the weather becomes warm.

Phlegm rheum that lies deep internally, fusing and binding and not being removed, was regarded by the ancients as the deep-seated root of dyspnea and wheezing. When it is stimulated by wind cold external evils, it will attack the lungs. When qi lifts the shoulders upward, this is known as panting. When sound comes from the throat, it is called wheezing. Because phlegm rheum is the deep-seated root of asthma, as long as it is retained and is not removed, spleen and kidney yang qi is therefore obstructed. This is the chief root and source of the complications of cardiopulmonary diseases. If superficial edema appears on the four limbs, head, and face and there is rapid breathing, it is necessary to prevent inversion desertion. It is advisable to send for a doctor at once.

Treatment based on pattern discrimination

A. Phlegm rheum cough

Main symptoms: Cough and abundant phlegm, white colored phlegm which is watery and mixed with foam, chest fullness and oppression, devitalized essence spirit, fear of cold, a white tongue with a slimy coating, and a soggy, slippery pulse.

Treatment principles: Warmly transform phlegm rheum, diffuse the lungs and transform stasis

Rx: Mix-fried Herba Ephedrae (*Ma Huang*), 6g, Sichuan Ramulus Cinnamomi (*Chuan Gui Zhi*), 6g, Rhizoma Atractylodis Macrocephalae (*Bai Zhu*), 6g, Radix Albus Paeoniae Lactiflorae (*Bai Shao*), 6g, Fructus Schizandrae Chinensis (*Wu Wei Zi*), 4.5g, dry Rhizoma Zingiberis (*Gan Jiang*), 2.4g, Herba Cum Radice Asari Seiboldi (*Xi Xin*), 3g, Rhizoma Pinelliae Ternatae (*Ban Xia*), 9g, mix-fried Radix Glycyrrhizae (*Zhi Gan Cao*), 2.4g, Sclerotium Poriae Cocos (*Fu Ling*), 9g, Radix Salviae Miltiorrhizae (*Dan Shen*), 12g, Fructus Zizyphi Jujubae (*Da Zao*), 5 pieces

B. Phelgm rheum cough & wheezing

Main Symptoms: Panting, shortness of breath, a low, weak coughing sound, bodily emaciation, spiritual fatigue. When cough and wheezing are severe, there is much exhalation and little inhalation, as if the breath cannot be continued. The tongue is pale and purplish with static patches. The pulse is soft and fine.

Treatment principles: Warm yang and transform rheum, quicken the blood and transform stasis

Rx: Sclerotium Poriae Cocos (*Fu Ling*), 9g, Ramulus Cinnamomi (*Gui Zhi*), 9g, dry Rhizoma Zingiberis (*Gan Jiang*), 3 grams, Fructus Schizandrae Chinensis (*Wu Wei Zi*), 6g, Rhizoma Atractylodis Macro-cephalae (*Bai Zhu*), 9g, mix-fried Radix Glycyrrhizae (*Zhi Gan Cao*), 4.5g, Rhizoma Pinelliae Ternatae (*Ban Xia*), 9g, mix-fried Flos Tussilaginis Farfarae (*Dong Hua*), 9g, Cortex Magnoliae Officinalis (*Chuan Po*), 6g, Fructus Perillae Frutescentis (*Su Zi*), 9g, Stalactitum (*E Guan Shi*), 30g, Radix Angelicae Sinensis (*Dang Gui*), 9g, Hirudo (*Shui Zhi*), 2.4g

C. Phlegm rheum internally stopping

Main symptoms: Coughing (*spittle*), chest fullness, phlegm like white foam, many bowlsful, shortness of breath, and rapid respiration. If severe, the patient is able to lie flat. The tongue is pale with a white coating. The pulse is wiry and slippery. This condition often persists over years and cannot be cured. It recurs whenever the patient meets with cold.

Treatment principles: Transport the spleen and transform phlegm, quicken the blood and transform stasis

Rx: Rhizoma Pinelliae Ternatae (*Ban Xia*), 9g, uncooked Rhizoma Zingiberis (*Sheng Jiang*), 3 slices, Semen Lepidii (*Ting Li Zi*), 9g, Semen Sinapis Albae (*Bai Jie Zi*), 9g, Sclerotium Poriae Cocos (*Fu Ling*), 9g, Radix Lateralis Praeparatus Aconiti Carmichaeli (*Fu Zi*), 9g, Rhizoma Atractylodis Macrocephalae (*Bai Zhu*), 9g, mix-fried Herba Ephedrae (*Ma Huang*), 9g, Herba Cum Radice Asari Seiboldi (*Xi Xin*), 4.5g, Exocarpium Citri Rubri (*Ju Hong*), 6g, Hirudo (*Shui Zhi*), 2.4g

Secret essentials

1. Phlegm rheum is invariably due to water rheum internally stopping with yang vacuity and yin congelation. The general outline for treating this is as follows: When it shines in the sky, dark clouds will spontaneously disperse. Therefore, use medicinals which mainly diffuse and warm yang. I like to use Aconite and Ephedra together to treat both the lungs and kidneys. This addresses both root and branch. Therefore, one can usually administer these medicinals in this disease.

2. Counterflow cough and panting and wheezing cannot be separated from the lungs, nor do they merely remain in the lungs. Because this disease tends to linger on, it will definitely produce stasis. If phlegm and stasis join and obstruct, then aside from warming and transforming, it is further necessary to transform stasis. In mild cases, Lignum Sappan

(*Su Mu*) and Radix Salviae Miltiorrhizae (*Dan Shen*) should be used. In severe cases, Hirudo (*Shui Zhi*) and Pollen Typhae (*Pu Huang*) should be used. Thus better effects may be obtained like one dotting the pupil in the eyeball of the painted dragon (which then comes to life and flies off the wall).

3. Take 250g of uncooked Rhizoma Zingiberis (*Sheng Jiang*), pound it into paste, and wring out its juice. Then put this in 90g of clear jelly, 4.5g of Resina Olibani (*Ru Xiang*), and 4.5g of Resina Myrrhae (*Mo Yao*). Bring to a boil, dissolve, and stir them evenly. Then again put in 6g of powdered Fructus Zanthoxyli Bungeani (*Chuan Jiao*), stir the ingredients evenly, spread them on heavy paper, and stick this gently on the acupoints *Da Zhui* (GV 14) and bilaterally on *Fei Shu* (Bl 13) and *Gao Huang* (Bl 43). After 3-5 days, remove this plaster. If there are blisters, prick them and prevent infection. This methods helps to satisfactorily treat phlegm rheum cough and wheezing and a chilly, icy feeling in the upper back.

4. Decoct together 30g of Semen Lepidii (*Ting Li Zi*) and 21 pieces of Fructus Zizyphi Jujubae (*Da Zao*). When the juice has boiled away, take out the Red Dates, remove their skin and kernels, and eat them for 3 successive days. This medicine dispels phlegm without damaging the righteous. It is generally effective for asthma patients who cannot lie down flat.

3. Diarrhea (*Xie Xie*)

If the stool is thin and loose, this is called discharge. If the stool is watery, this is known as drainage.[1] Clinically, these appear simultaneously. Thus it is generally called discharge and drainage or diarrhea. If the feces are mixed with water and grain, clear and turbid are not

---

[1] *Xie xie* is a compound term which means diarrhea. It is made up of one word which means discharge and another word which means drainage.

separated. It may also be accompanied by abdominal pain or abdominal distension.

Disease causes, disease mechanisms

The *Nei Jing (Inner Classic)* says, "Excessive dampness produces diarrhea." This saying strikes the point. The disease mechanism of diarrhea is the loss of normalcy of the spleen and stomach's transportation and transformation and the inability of the intestinal tract to open and close. The *Jing Yue Quan Shu (The Complete Writings of Jing-yue)* states:

> If one's drinking and eating are undisciplined and their lifestyle is not timed (*i.e.*, is irregular), this will result in the spleen and stomach suffering damage. Water will then produce dampness, and grain will also become stagnant. The qi of essence flourishing is not able to be transported and transformed. These combine to form filth which descends and downbears. Thus drainage is uninhibited.

This analysis is just so. However, if diarrhea lasts a long time and is not cured, static blood must necessarily obstruct in the hidden corners of the intestine, and this should not be neglected.

Treatment based on pattern discrimination

A. Cold damp diarrhea

Main symptoms: Slight abdominal pain, clear, watery stools, bodily heaviness, fatigue, reduced appetite, chest oppression, no thirst in the mouth, a white, slimy tongue coating, and a mostly soggy, relaxed (*i.e.*, retarded) pulse

Treatment principles: Warm the center and scatter cold, transform dampness and harmonize the blood

Rx: Radix Codonopsis Pilosulae (*Dang Shen*), 9g, Rhizoma Atracty-lodis (*Cang Zhu*), 9g, Rhizoma Atractylodis Macrocephalae (*Bai Zhu*), 9g, Sclerotium Poriae Cocos (*Fu Ling*), 9g, blast-fried Rhizoma Zingiberis (*Pao Jiang*), 4.5g, Fructus Perillae Frutecentis (*Zi Su*), 9g, Radix Et Rhizoma Notopterygii (*Qiang Huo*), 9g, roasted Radix Ledebouriellae Sesloidis (*Fang Feng*), 9g, Pericarpium Citri Reticulatae (*Chen Pi*), 6g, Massa Medica Fermentata (*Cha Qu*), 9g, Radix Ligustici Wallichii (*Chuan Xiong*), 4.5g

B. Damp heat diarrhea

Main symptoms: This is mostly seen between summer and autumn (in China). Abdominal pain accompanies diarrhea. There is burning heat around the anus. The feces are yellowish brown. Urination is short and red. There is heart vexation and oral thirst. The tongue coating is yellow and slimy, and the pulse is slippery and rapid.

Treatment principles: Clear and transform dampness and heat, transport the spleen and disperse stasis

Rx: Radix Puerariae (*Ge Gen*), 9g, Radix Scutellariae Baicalensis (*Huang Qin*), 9g, Rhizoma Coptidis Chinensis (*Huang Lian*), 3g, Flos Capsellae Bursa-pastoris (*Ji Cai Hua*), 30g, Semen Raphani Sativi (*Lai Fu Zi*), 9g, Rhizoma Pinelliae Ternatae (*Ban Xia*), 9g, Sclerotium Poriae Cocos (*Fu Ling*), 9g, roasted Radix Saussureae Seu Vladimiriae (*Mu Xiang*), 4.5g, Shi Xiao San (Sudden Smile Powder, *i.e.*, Feces Trogop-terori Seu Pteromi [*Wu Ling Zhi*] & Pollen Typhae [*Pu Huang*]), 9g, wrapped during decoction, Massa Medica Fermentata (*Cha Qu*), 9g, Pericarpium Citri Reticulatae (*Chen Pi*), 6g

C. Spleen vacuity diarrhea

Main symptoms: A sallow yellow complexion, no thought for food and drink, spiritual fatigue and exhaustion, hands and feet clear and chilly, diarrhea with untransformed grain, a pale tongue with a white coating, and a soggy, weak pulse

Treatment principles: Boost the qi and upbear yang, warm the center and quicken the blood

Rx: Radix Astragali Membranacei (*Huang Qi*), 15g, Radix Codonopsis Pilosulae (*Dang Shen*), 9g, mix-fried Radix Glycyrrhizae (*Zhi Gan Cao*), 3g, Pericarpium Citri Reticulatae (*Chen Pi*), 6g, mix-fried Rhizoma Cimicifugae (*Sheng Ma*), 9g, Radix Bupleuri (*Chai Hu*), 9g, Rhizoma Atractylodis (*Cang Zhu*), 9g, roasted Radix Saussureae Seu Vladimiriae (*Mu Xiang*), 6g, Radix Ligustici Wallichii (*Chuan Xiong*), 6g, uncooked Rhizoma Zingiberis (*Sheng Jiang*), 3 slices, Fructus Zizyphi Jujubae (*Da Zao*), 5 pieces

Note: If this formula is not effective, one can add *Ge Xia Zhu Yu Tang* (Below the Diaphragm Dispel Stasis Decoction): Stir-fried Feces Tropgopterori Seu Pteromi (*Wu Ling Zhi*), Radix Ligustici Wallichii (*Chuan Xiong*), Cortex Radicis Moutan (*Dan Pi*), Radix Rubrus Paeoniae Lactiflorae (*Chi Shao*), Radix Linderae Strychnifoliae (*Wu Yao*), Rhizoma Corydalis Yanhusuo (*Yan Hu Suo*), 6g @, Radix Glycyrrhizae (*Gan Cao*), 3g, Radix Angelicae Sinensis (*Dang Gui*), Semen Pruni Persicae (*Tao Ren*), Flos Carthami Tinctorii (*Hong Hua*), 9g @, Rhizoma Cyperi Rotundi (*Xiang Fu*), Fructus Citri Seu Ponciri (*Zhi Qiao*), 4.5g @

D. Kidney vacuity diarrhea

Main symptoms: Fifth watch (*i.e.*, daybreak) diarrhea, abdominal pain, intestinal rumbling, quiet after defecation, cold body, chilled limbs, low back and knee soreness and weakness, a pale tongue with a white coating, and a deep, fine pulse

Treatment principles: Warm the kidneys and fortify the spleen, transform stasis and stop diarrhea

Rx: Radix Codonopsis Pilosulae (*Dang Shen*), 9g, Sclerotium Poriae Cocos (*Fu Ling*), 9g, blackened Radix Lateralis Praeparatus Aconiti Carmichaeli (*Fu Zi*), 9g, Rhizoma Atractylodis Macrocephalae (*Bai Zhu*), 9g, blast-fried Rhizoma Zingiberis (*Pao Jiang*), 3g, Semen Trigonellae Foeni-graeci (*Hu Lu Ba*), 9g, Fructus Alpiniae Oxyphyllae (*Yi Zhi Ren*), 9g, Cortex Cinnamomi (*Guan Gui*), 4.5g, Fructus Chaenomelis Lagenariae (*Mu Gua*), 9g, *Shi Xiao San* (Sudden Smile Powder, *i.e.*, Feces Trogopterori Seu Pteromi [*Wu Ling Zhi*] & Pollen Typhae [*Pu Huang*]), 9g, wrapped during decoction

Secret essentials

1. In old peoples' bodies, downbearing is excessive and upbearing is scanty, scattering is excessive and gathering is scanty. Therefore, it is not appropriate to attack too much. In treating the root, one should mainly fortify the spleen and warm the kidneys, while in treating the branch, dispelling cold and transforming stasis should be used as aids. For the former, *Fu Zi Li Zhong Tang* (Aconite Rectify the Center Decoction) should be administered, while for the latter, one should use Wang Qing-ren's *Ge Xia Zhu Yu Tang* (Below the Diaphragm Dispel Stasis Decoction). These decoctions usually prove efficacious. Treating diarrhea by transforming stasis was Wang Qing-ren's favorite method. According to my own clinical experience, this method has merit.

2. If the emotions and orientation run counter to harmony, liver qi will counterflow transversely, attacking the spleen and stomach. In this case, there is diarrhea and abdominal pain with the simultaneous appearance of complaining and lack of cheer. For this, it is appropriate to use *Tong Xie Yao Fang* (Essential Formula for Painful Diarrhea) combined with *Si Ni San* (Four Counterflows Powder): Radix Ledebouriellae Sesloidis (*Fang Feng*), 6g, Rhizoma Atractylodis Macrocephalae (*Bai Zhu*), 9g,

Radix Albus Paeoniae Lactiflorae (*Bai Shao*), 9g, Pericarpium Citri Reticulatae (*Chen Pi*), 6g, Radix Bupleuri (*Chai Hu*), 6g, Fructus Immaturus Citri Seu Ponciri (*Zhi Shi*), 9g, Radix Glycyrrhizae (*Gan Cao*), 3g, plus Fructus Citri Sacrodactylis (*Fo Shou Gan*), 6g, and Flos Hemerocallis (*Yi Nan Hua*), 9g, as messengers, this gets good results.

3. The ready-made remedy *Xiang Lian Wan* (Saussurea & Coptis Pills) is an ancient formula for the treatment of dysentery. I have used this remedy in treating gastrointestinal indigestion and diarrhea in the early stage. Its therapeutic effect is also satisfactory. For watery stool, *Huo Xiang Zheng Qi Wan* (Agastaches Righteous Qi Pills) should be administered. For enduring diarrhea which will not stop or if the patient feels chilly pain within their abdomen, results may be observed after administering 3-5 doses of *Chun Yang Zheng Qi Wan* (Pure Yang Righteous Qi Pills).

4. Constipation (*Bian Bi*)

Constipation refers to scanty fluids and moisture in the intestines. This leads to loss of their function of conduction. Zhang Jie-gu said:

> Constipation in the viscera and bowels cannot be treated without discrimination. There is vacuity constipation. There is repletion constipation. There is wind constipation. There is qi constipation. There is chill constipation. There is heat constipation. There is fluid and humor dryness in the elderly. There is loss of blood, emission of perspiration, and disinhibition of urination in postpartum women and failure of restoration of qi and blood after illness. All these may cause constipation.

This clearly explains that the occurrence of constipation has various types and one cannot use the same method of treatment on all of these. In the elderly, there commonly appear dry heat, qi stagnation, vacuity constipation, and chill which are differentiated below.

Disease causes, disease mechanisms

Accumulation of heat in the intestines and stomach is mostly due to constitutional yang exuberance or to overeating acrid, peppery, thick flavors. These lead to heat toxins becoming exuberant internally. These consume and damage fluids and humors. Thus the intestinal tract is dry and astringed. If the qi mechanism is depressed and stagnant, this is mostly due to worry and thought, prolonged sitting, or lack of motion. This leads to loss of normalcy in free flow and downbearing as well as to internal stoppage of waste matter. In the elderly, qi, blood, and yin fluids are deficient. If qi is vacuous, there is no force for propulsion, and if blood is vacuous, there is no water on which the ship can travel. Taxation beyond limit, excessive perspiration, and undisciplined bedroom affairs may all also cause vacuity constipation. True yang is also typically insufficient in the elderly. In that case, yin cold congeals and binds, there is lack of qi for warming and the steaming transformation of fluids. Thus the function of conduction may lose its duty and may bring about chill constipation.

Treatment based on pattern discrimination

A. Dry heat constipation

Main symptoms: Dry, bound stool, short, red urination, vexatious thirst, bad breath, abdominal distention, fullness, and oppression, a red tongue with a dry, yellow coating, and a slippery, rapid pulse

Treatment principles: Clear heat and moisten the intestines, quicken the blood and conduct stagnation

Rx: Radix Et Rhizoma Rhei (*Da Huang*), 6g, Fructus Immaturus Citri Seu Ponciri (*Zhi Shi*), 9g, Semen Pruni Persicae (*Tao Ren*), 9g, Radix Trichosanthis Kirlowii (*Hua Fen*), 9g, Pericarpium Arecae Catechu (*Fu Pi*), 9g, Radix Scutellariae Baicalensis (*Huang Qin*), 9g, Rhizoma

Phragmitis Communis (*Lu Gen*), 30g, Radix Angelicae Sinensis (*Dang Gui*), 9g, powdered Mirabilitum (*Yuan Ming*), 9g, dissolved after the other ingredients are decocted

B. Qi stagnation constipation

Main symptoms: Dry or bound stools, defecation not easy, frequent burping, fullness and oppression in the hypochondral region, a red tongue with white coating, and a wiry pulse

Treatment principles: Normalize the qi and resolve depression, quicken the blood and conduct stagnation

Rx: Radix Linderae Strychnifoliae (*Wu Yao*), 6g, uncooked Rhizoma Cyperi Rotundi (*Xiang Fu*), 9g, Lignum Aquilariae Agallochae (*Chen Xiang*), 1.5, Fructus Immaturus Citri Seu Ponciri (*Zhi Shi*), 9g, Semen Arecae Catechu (*Bing Lang*), 9g, wine-processed Radix Et Rhizoma Rhei (*Da Huang*), 6g, Semen Pruni Persicae (*Tao Ren*), 9g, Radix Angelicae Sinensis (*Dang Gui*), 9g, Semen Biotae Orientalis (*Bai Zi Ren*), 9g, Pericarpium Viridis Citri Reticulatae (*Qing Pi*), 6g

C. Qi stagnation & vacuity constipation

Main symptoms: A lusterless complexion, a willingness to defecate yet no force to do so, dizziness, vertigo, sweating, heart palpitations, shortness of breath, disinclination to speak, a pale tongue with a white coating, and fine, weak pulse

Treatment principles: Boost the qi and nourish yin, quicken the blood and moisten dryness

Rx: Herba Cistanchis (*Cong Rong*), 9g, Radix Achyranthis Bidentatae (*Niu Xi*), 9g, Radix Angelicae Sinensis (*Dang Gui*), 9g, Semen Pruni Persicae (*Tao Ren*), 9g, Lignum Aquilariae Agallochae (*Chen Xiang*),

2.4g, uncooked Radix Polygoni Multiflori (*Shou Wu*), 15g, Semen Pruni (*Yu Li Ren*), 9g, Semen Cannabis Sativae (*Huo Ma Ren*), 9g, Herba Cynomorii Songarici (*Suo Yang*), 9g

D. Yang vacuity chill constipation

Main symptoms: A clear, white complexion, lack of warmth in the hands and feet, lower and upper back chill and heaviness, urination clear and long, one bowel movement per week, some slight discomfort in the abdomen, a pale tongue with a white coating, and a deep, slow pulse

Treatment principles: Warm, moisten, and free the stools, quicken the blood and transform stasis

Rx: *Ban Liu Wan* (Half Sulfur Pills), 30 pills each time, 2 time per day, or *Fu Gui Ba Wei Wan* (Aconite & Cinnamon Eight Flavors Pills), 9g each time, 2 times per day.

Secret essentials

1. If the fluids and humors are vacuous or after yin has already been damaged, then it is not proper to use only the precipitating method. In such cases, it is appropriate to use "supplementing medicinals as the root while also using moving and draining medicinals." For instance, Radix Scrophulariae Ningpoensis (*Xuan Shen*), Tuber Ophiopogonis Japonicae (*Mai Dong*), Semen Negrum Sesami Indici (*Hei Zhi Ma*), uncooked Radix Polygoni Multiflori (*Shou Wu*), uncooked Radix Rehmanniae (*Sheng Di*), Radix Achyranthis Bidentatae (*Niu Xi*), 12g @ should be decocted in water and administered so as to increase the water on which the ship can travel.

2. In case of senile habitual constipation, Semen Pruni Persicae (*Tao Ren*), 9g, Radix Angelicae Sinensis (*Dang Gui*), 9g, Semen Cannabis

Sativae (*Huo Ma Ren*), 9g, Semen Pruni (*Yu Li Ren*), 9g, and Semen Cassiae Torae (*Jue Ming Zi*), 30g, should be decocted in water and administered in order to quicken the blood and free the secreted miraculously.

3. To the various formulas above, 15 grams of uncooked Radix Asteris Tatarici (*Zi Wan*) should be added to increase the therapeutic effect. This is because the lungs and large intestine are joined in a mutual exterior and interior relationship.

5. Strangury

The *Chao Shi Bing Yuan (Master Chao's Origins of Disease)* states:

> Kidney vacuity leads to polyuria. Bladder heat leads to the precipitation of urine being astringent. If urination is numerous yet astringent, this leads to dribbling and dripping which is not appropriate. This is called strangury.

Strangury means that the urination is numerous (*i.e.*, frequent), short, and astringent. During urination, one may also feel pricking pain, and they are unable to urinate completely. The lower abdomen is tense or pain may extend to the low back and abdomen. There are five types of strangury, namely, stone strangury, qi strangury, blood strangury, unctuous strangury, and taxation strangury.

Disease causes, disease mechanisms

The chief cause of strangury is damp heat accompanied by stasis brewing and binding in the lower burner. If damp heat persists for a long time, within the urination there will bind gravel and stones. This is called stone strangury. If damp heat obstructs congests and obstructs, it will damage the network vessels. Blood will be forced to move recklessly. This is called blood strangury. If qi stagnates and is not diffused, urination becomes astringent, and there is terminal dribbling which does not stop. This is called qi strangury. If damp heat lingers for many days, the urine will become fatty and slimy like paste. The clear and turbid are not separated, and the urination becomes astringent and painful. This is called unctuous strangury. If the condition endures and is not cured, if it occurs when the patient feels tired due to taxation, and if the urine dribbles endlessly with falling and distention in the lower abdomen and low back and knee soreness and weakness, this is called taxation strangury. The symptoms of these various types of strangury are not all the same. However, the main cause of this disease is damp heat stasis and obstruction. At first, it is usually a pattern of evil repletion. In enduring disease, repletion transmutes into vacuity. There may also be patterns of vacuity mixed with repletion.

Treatment based on pattern discrimination

A. Stone strangury

Main symptoms: Urine mixed with gravel and stones, urination difficult and astringent or suddenly interrupted, possible piercing pain and urgency, wringing low back pain radiating to the lower abdomen and external genitalia, and a reddish tongue. If the disease is enduring, the tongue may be pale. Its coating is thin and yellow. The pulse is wiry and rapid.

Treatment principles: Free strangury and expel stones, clear heat and transform stasis

Rx: Caulis Akebiae Mutong (*Mu Tong*), 9g, Herba Dianthi (*Qu Mai*), 9g, Herba Plantaginis (*Che Qian Cao*), 30g, Talcum (*Hua Shi*), 9g, rootlets of Radix Glycyrrhizae (*Gan Cao Xiao*), 3g, Radix Et Rhizoma Rhei (*Da Huang*), 9g, Herba Pyrossiae (*Shi Wei*), 15g, Semen Abutilonis Seu Malvae (*Dong Kui Zi*), 9g, Rhizoma Curcumae Zedoariae (*E Zhu*), 9g, Herba Desmodii Seu Lysimachiae (*Jin Yin Cao*), 30g, Spora

Lygodii (*Hai Jin Sha*), 9g, Endothelium Corneum Gigeriae Galli (*Ji Nei Jin*), 9g, blast-fried Squama Manitis Pentadactylis (*Shan Jia*), 6g

B. Blood strangury

Main symptoms: Hot, astringent urination with pricking pain, purplish urine or possible blood clots, aching, pain, fullness, and urgency, vexatious heat in the heart, a red tongue tip with a yellow coating, and a rapid, forceful pulse

Treatment principles: Cool and quicken the blood, disinhibit dampness and free strangury

Rx: Rhizoma Anemarrhenae (*Zhi Mu*), 9g, Cortex Phellodendri (*Huang Bai*), 9g, uncooked Pollen Typhae (*Pu Huang*), 9g, wrapped during decoction, Radix Viticis Pentaphyllae (*Wu Liam Mei*), 15g, Radix Cyathulae (*Chuan Niu Xi*), 9g, Spora Lygodii (*Hai Jin Sha*), 9g, Herba Ecliptae Prostratae (*Han Lian Cao*), 9g, uncooked Nodus Nelumbinis Nuciferae (*Ou Jie*), 9g, Semen Pruni Persicae (*Tao Ren*), 9g, Radix Rubrus Paeoniae Lactiflorae (*Chi Shao*), 9g, Rhizoma Imperatae Cylindricae (*Bai Mao Gen*), 30g

C. Qi strangury

Main symptoms: Astringent, painful urination, lower abdomen fullness and urgency, dribbling and dripping, inhibited urination, terminal dribbling which does not stop, a bluish purple tongue, and a deep, wiry pulse

Treatment principles: Rectify the qi and harmonize the blood, free strangury and disinhibit urination

Rx: Powdered Lignum Aquilariae Agallochae (*Chen Xiang*), 1.5g, added after the other ingredients are decocted, Herba Pyrossiae (*Shi*

Wei), 15g, Talcum (*Hua Shi*), 9g, tails of Radix Angelicae Sinensis (*Gui Wei*), 9g, Radix Rubrus Paeoniae Lactiflorae (*Chi Shao*), 9g, Semen Abutilonis Seu Malvae (*Dong Kui Zi*), 9g, Radix Glycyrrhizae (*Gan Cao*), 3g, Semen Vaccariae Segetalis (*Wang Bu Liu Xing*), 9g, Pericarpium Viridis Citri Reticulatae (*Qing Pi*), 9g, Fructus Foeniculi Vulgaris (*Xiao Hui Xiang*), 2.4g, Radix Linderae Strychnifoliae (*Wu Yao*), 9g, Rhizoma Sparganii (*San Leng*), 9g, Curcumae Zedoariae (*E Zhu*), 9g

D. Unctuous strangury

Main symptoms: Cloudy, turbid urine like rice-washing water, slime floating on the top like fat, and heat, astringency, and aching and pain in the urinary tract. If the symptoms linger and endure, the body become progressively emaciated. There is dizziness and lack of strength, low back and knee soreness and weakness, a pale tongue with a slimy coating, and a fine, forceless pulse.

Treatment principles: Transform stasis and rectify dampness, divide the clear and discharge the turbid

Rx: Rhizoma Dioscoreae Hypoglaucae (*Bi Xie*), 9g, Rhizoma Acori Graminei (*Chang Pu*), 9g, Radix Linderae Strychnifoliae (*Wu Yao*), 9g, Rhizoma Cimicifugae (*Sheng Ma*), 6g, Fructus Trigonellae Foeni-graeci (*Hu Lu Ba*), 9g, Herba Pyrossiae (*Shi Wei*), 15g, blast-fried Squama Manitis Pentadactylis (*Shan Jia*), 9g, uncooked Pollen Typhae (*Pu Huang*), 9g, Rhizoma Curcumae Zedoariae (*E Zhu*), 9g, vinegar stir-fried Radix Bupleuri (*Chai Hu*), 6g, *Zi Shen Tong Guan Wan* (Enrich the Kidneys & Open the Barrier Pills),[2] 9g, wrapped during decoction

E. Taxation strangury

Main symptoms: Redness and astringency of the urinary flow not

---

[2] This formula is composed of: Cortex Phellodendri (*Huang Bai*), Rhizoma Anemarrhenae (*Zhi Mu*), and Cortex Cinnamomi (*Rou Gui*).

severe, aching and pain with discharge not pronounced, a lingering disease course, sometimes better, sometimes worse, occurs on taxation, endless dribbling of urination, a pale tongue, and a fine pulse

Treatment principles: Supplement the kidneys and free strangury, quicken the blood and transform stasis

Rx: Prepared Radix Rehmanniae (*Shu Di*), 20g, Cortex Eucommiae Ulmoidis (*Du Zhong*), 9g, Ramus Loranthi Seu Visci (*Sang Ji Sheng*), 15g, Radix Dipsaci (*Chuan Duan*), 9g, Fructus Lycii Chinensis (*Qi Zi*), 9g, Cornu Degelatinum Cervi (*Lu Jiao Shuang*), 9g, powdered Radix Pseudoginseng (*Shen San Qi*), 1.5g, added after the other ingredients are decocted, Fructus Foeniculi Vulgaris (*Xiao Hui Xiang*), 2.4g, Rhizoma Alismatis (*Ze Xie*), 15g, Radix Achyranthis Bidentatae (*Niu Xi*), 9g, Semen Plantaginis (*Che Qian Zi*), 9g

Secret essentials

1. If the above method proves ineffectual for stone strangury, then the flow should be facilitated by warming and opening. In that case, 6g of Radix Lateralis Praeparatus Aconiti Carmichaeli (*Fu Zi*) can be added into this formula. Thus when qi obtains yang's assistance, accumulated stones can be precipitated.

2. If stone strangury endures and cannot be cured, then it is appropriate to use heavy amounts of quickening the blood and transforming stasis medicinals, such as Semen Vaccariae Segetalis (*Wang Bu Liu Xing*), Rhizoma Sparganii (*San Leng*), Rhizoma Curcumae Zedoariae (*E Zhu*), blast-fried Squama Manitis Pentadactylis (*Shan Jia*), Radix Cyathulae (*Chuan Niu Xi*) and Flos Carthami Tinctorii (*Hong Hua*). The above two methods are able to both propel the bound stones and to expel such disinhibited bound stones outside.

3. In the formula for unctuous strangury, 1.5g of Semen Momordicae Cochinensis (*Mu Bie*) should be added to the decoction. (It should not

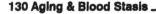

be swallowed down but is only able to be decocted as an ingredient). This may improve the short-term therapeutic effect.

6. Impotence (*Yang Wei*)

Impotence means that, before the arrival of a male's normal decline in sexual function, the penis becomes flaccid and weak and cannot become erect. There is lack of erection during intercourse or, if there is intercourse, the penis is not hard.

Disease causes, disease mechanisms

Most discussions of impotence begin with sexual overindulgence. This leads to essence qi debility and exhaustion. However, in no small number of cases, it may also be caused by worry and anxiety which damage the liver as well as by qi stagnation and blood stasis. The *Nei Jing (Inner Classic)* states:

> Thinking and thinking without límit but not being able to obtain these desires, lascivious thoughts manifest externally and one's entry into the bedroom is too much. Thus the ancestral sinews becomes slack and loose, and this produces sinew atony and white turbidity.

It also says, "Sinew atony is mainly associated internally with the liver." However, its disease cause is not solely confined to this. It is also closely related to the essence spirit as described above.

Treatment based on pattern discrimination

A. Worry and anxiety damaging the liver

Main symptoms: Essence spirit bitter and oppressed, timidity and excessive suspicions, fright and fear, impotence occurring before entering the bedroom, a purple tongue, and a wiry pulse

Treatment principles: Course and rectify liver depression, transform stasis and open the network vessels

Rx: Radix Bupleuri (*Chai Hu*), 6g, Semen Allii Tuberosi (*Jiu Cai Zi*), 9g, Radix Achyranthis Bidentatae (*Niu Xi*), 4.5g, Radix Angelicae Sinensis (*Dang Gui*), 9g, uncooked Radix Rehmanniae (*Sheng Di*), 12g, Radix Ligustici Wallichii (*Chuan Xiong*), 6g, Radix Rubrus Paeoniae Lactiflorae (*Chi Shao*), 9g, Fructus Citri Seu Ponciri (*Zhi Qiao*), 6g, Radix Glycyrrhizae (*Gan Cao*), 3g, Flos Carthami Tinctorii (*Hong Hua*), 9g, Semen Pruni Persicae (*Tao Ren*), 9g, Radix Platycodi Grandiflori (*Jie Geng*), 4.5g, Fructus Cnidii Monnieri (*She Chuang Zi*), 9g

B. Kidney essence deficiency detriment

Main symptoms: Somber white complexion, dizziness and vertigo, essence spirit withering and wilting, low back and knee soreness and weakness, lack of erection during intercourse, a pale tongue with a white coating, and a deep, fine, forceless pulse

Treatment principles: Boost the qi and nourish the essence, quicken the blood and supplement the kidneys

Rx: Prepared Radix Rehmanniae (*Shu Di*), 24g, Semen Cuscutae (*Tu Si Zi*), 9g, Radix Morindae Officinalis (*Ba Ji Tian*), 9g, Semen Trigonellae Foeni-graeci (*Hu Lu Ba*), 9g, Rhizoma Curculiginis Orchoidis (*Xian Mao*), 9g, Herba Epimedii (*Xian Ling Pi*), 9g, Cortex Eucommiae Ulmoidis (*Du Zhong*), 9g, Fructus Lycii Chinensis (*Qi Zi*), 9g, Radix Angelicae Sinensis (*Dang Gui*), 9g, Cornu Cervi (*Lu Jiao Pian*), 9g, Fluoritum (*Zhi Shi Ying*), 30g, Semen Allii Tuberosi (*Jiu Cai Zi*), 9g

C. Heart & kidneys both damaged

Main symptoms: Heart palpitations, easy fear, heart vexation, loss of sleep, dizziness, low back soreness, premature discharge during intercourse or impotence, a thin, slimy tongue coating, and a fine, slippery pulse.

Treatment principles: Boost the kidneys and quicken the blood, nourish the heart and quiet the spirit

Rx: Semen Cuscutae (*Tu Si Zi*), 9g, Rhizoma Cibotii Barometz (*Gou Ji*), 9g, Herba Cynomorii Songarici (*Suo Yang*), 9g, Rhizoma Curculiginis Orchoidis (*Xian Mao*), 9g, mix-fried Radix Polygalae Tenuifoliae (*Yuan Zhi*), 9g, mix-fried Plastrum Testudinis (*Gui Ban*), 15g, Cortex Eucommiae Ulmoidis (*Du Zhong*), 9g, Herba Cistanchis (*Cong Rong*), 9g, Radix Salviae Miltiorrhizae (*Dan Shen*), 15g, Radix Rubrus Paeoniae Lactiflorae (*Chi Shao*), 9g, Flos Carthami Tinctorii (*Hong Hua*), 9g

Secret essentials

1. Impotence is one of the symptoms of senility. Therefore, the elderly should not conceal this symptom when they consult their physician. Even if one is over 80 years of age and their essence and blood are already debilitated and their ancestral sinew is loose, if one regularly takes *Liu Wei Di Huang Wan* (Six Flavors Rehmannia Pills), this will nourish yin and fulfil the essence. Take 9g each time, 2 times per day.

2. Impotence is a pattern associated with the liver channel. It is often seen when the heart is laden with worry. Liver qi becomes depressed and binds. Qi becomes stagnant and the blood becomes static. Therefore, one should not neglect to discriminate between vacuity and repletion and recklessly use supplementing, boosting, securing, and containing. In that case, the more one supplements, the more stagnation there will be, and the more one secures, the more it drips. Therefore, in such cases, I like to administer *Xue Fu Zhu Yu Tang* (Blood Mansion Dispel Stasis Decoction): Radix Bupleuri (*Chai Hu*), 6g, Radix Ligustici Wallichii (*Chuan Xiong*), 6g, Radix Angelicae Sinensis (*Dang Gui*), 9g, Radix Rubrus Paeoniae Lactiflorae (*Chi Shao*), 9g, Semen

Pruni Persicae (*Tao Ren*), 9g, uncooked Radix Rehmanniae (*Sheng Di*), 12g, Fructus Citri Seu Ponciri (*Zhi Qiao*), 5g, Radix Achyranthis Bidentatae (*Niu Xi*), 6g, Radix Glycyrrhizae (*Gan Cao*), 3g, Radix Platycodi Grandiflori (*Jie Geng*), 5g, Flos Carthami Tinctorii (*Hong Hua*), 9g, plus Fructus Cnidii Monnieri (*She Chuang Zi*), 9g, and Semen Allii Tuberosi (*Jiu Cai Zi*), 9g. The effect is quite satisfactory. Because there is a sufficiency of yin around the genitalia, cases of qi stagnation and blood stasis are quite numerous, and it is not all right to confine treatment of this disease merely to one single point, namely, supplementing the kidneys and strengthening yang.

3. Impotence may also be caused by effulgent ministerial fire. Thus the penis may become erect but is not able to fight. Such patients should take *Zhi Bai Di Huang Wan* (Anemarrhena & Phellodendron Rehmannia Pills), 9g each time, 2 times per day. If impotence is caused by downward flow of damp heat, the penis will become flaccid and soft and the scrotum has a foul odor. In this case, use *San Miao Wan* (Three Wonders Pills), 9g each time, 2 tikes per day. This treatment is usually effective.

7. Tinnitus (*Er Ming*) & Deafness (*Er Long*)

The ears are the external portals of the kidneys. The chapter titled "Vessels Delimited" in the *Ling Shu (Spiritual Pivot)* states:

> Kidney qi flows freely to the ears. If the kidneys are harmonious, the ears are able to hear the five sounds.

Hearing may be abnormal, as if one hears the chirping of a cicada or the roar of the tide. This is called tinnitus. If qi closes and one cannot hear, that is called deafness. Tinnitus may be accompanied by deafness, and, in many cases, deafness develops from tinnitus.

Disease causes, disease mechanisms

If kidney qi has been vacuous for some time, wind evils may invade from outside and harass the clear portals. The patient may suddenly hear nothing. This is called sudden deafness. If evil and righteous struggle with each other, evil qi may stop and stagnate in the pathways of the ear. In that case, the ringing sound will not stop. If one's emotions are depressed, liver qi may harass internally and may travel along the channels upward to the ears. Thus there may be tinnitus, vexation and agitation, and easy anger. If phlegm dampness is exuberant internally, these may mist the clear portals. Then there may be either tinnitus like the chirping of cicadas or qi closes and nothing can be heard. If mixed with stasis, qi will lose its moistening and nourishing and may also cause deafness. This may also be due vacuity and deficiency or essence blood insufficiency. The channels and vessels lose their construction and are not able to supply these above. Thus dizziness and hardness of hearing may appear. In addition, yang qi may be devitalized and so channel qi may be empty and vacuous. Clear yang does not unfold and cannot fill above. All these causes manifest as loss of auditory acuity.

Treatment based on pattern discrimination

A. Wind evils externally invading

Main symptoms: Sudden tinnitus, sudden deafness, headache, aversion to wind, possible fever, joint soreness and pain, possible itching and pain in the ear, a floating, rapid pulse, and a thin, white tongue coating

Treatment principles: Course wind and resolve the exterior, quicken the blood and nourish the portals

Rx: Herba Schizonepetae Tenuifoliae (*Jing Jie*), 9g, Radix Ledebouriellae Sesloidis (*Fang Feng*), 9g, Flos Chrysanthemi Morifolii (*Ju Hua*), 9g, Rhizoma Acori Graminei (*Chang Pu*), 9g, Medulla Tetrapanacis Papyriferi (*Tong Cao*), 3g, Radix Rubrus Paeoniae Lactiflorae (*Chi Shao*), 9g, Cortex Radicis Moutan (*Dan Pi*), 9g, Radix Salviae Miltiorrhizae (*Dan Shen*), 9g, Flos Lonicerae Japonicae (*Yin Hua*), 9g, Fructus Forsythiae Suspensae (*Lian Qiao*), 9g, Radix Isatidis Seu Baphicacanthi (*Ban Lan Gen*), 15g

B. Liver/gallbladder fire exuberance

Main symptoms: Tinnitus, episodic loss of auditory acuity, headache, a red face, a bitter taste in the mouth, dry throat, heart vexation, easy anger, evening sleep not quiet, constipation, a red tongue with a yellow coating, and a wiry, rapid, and forceful pulse

Treatment principles: Clear the liver and discharge fire, quicken the blood and transform stasis

Rx: Radix Gentianae Scabrae (*Long Dan Cao*), 9g, Fructus Gardeniae Jasminoidis (*Shan Zhi*), 9g, Rhizoma Coptidis Chinensis (*Huang Lian*), 3g, Radix Et Rhizoma Rhei (*Da Huang*), 9g, Aloe (*Lu Hui*), 9g, Radix Bupleuri (*Chai Hu*), 9g, Radix Rubrus Paeoniae Lactiflorae (*Chi Shao*), 9g, Caulis Akebiae Mutong (*Mu Tong*), 6g, Rhizoma Alismatis (*Ze Xie*), 9g, Semen Plantaginis (*Che Qian Zi*), 9g, Sclerotium Rubrum Poriae Cocos (*Chi Ling*), 9g, Cortex Radicis Moutan (*Dan Pi*), 9g

C. Phlegm fire depression & binding

Main symptoms: Tinnitus like the chirping of cicadas, occasional blockage and obstruction similar to deafness, chest oppression, excessive phlegm, a thin, yellow, slimy tongue coating, and a slippery, rapid pulse

Treatment principles: Clear the qi and transform phlegm, quicken the blood and open the portals

Rx: Radix Scutellariae Baicalensis (*Huang Qin*), 9g, Radix Bupleuri (*Chai Hu*), 9g, Rhizoma Coptidis Chinensis (*Huang Lian*), 3g, Fructus Citri Seu Ponciri (*Zhi Qiao*), 9g, Rhizoma Acori Graminei (*Chang Pu*), 9g, Lapis Chloriti (*Qing Meng Shi*), 15g, Rhizoma Pinelliae Ternatae (*Ban Xia*), 9g, bile(-processed) Rhizoma Arisaematis (*Dan Xing*), 6g, Pericarpium Citri Reticulatae (*Chen Pi*), 6g, Radix Rubrus Paeoniae Lactiflorae (*Chi Shao*), 15g, Succus Bambusae (*Zhu Li*), 1 shoot, Succus Rhizomatis Zingiberis (*Jiang Zhi*), 10 drops

D. Stasis obstructing the ancestral vessel

Main symptoms: Deafness as if obstructed, a dark, black complexion, ear wax mixed with old blood, a choppy pulse, and a purple tongue with a slimy coating

Treatment principles: Clear the portals and quicken the blood, transform stasis and open the network vessels

Rx: Radix Rubrus Paeoniae Lactiflorae (*Bai Shao*), 9g, Radix Rubrus Paeoniae Lactiflorae (*Chi Shao*), 9g, Semen Pruni Persicae (*Tao Ren*), 9g, Flos Carthami Tinctorii (*Hong Hua*), 9g, Radix Angelicae Sinensis (*Dang Gui*), 9g, Radix Salviae Miltiorrhizae (*Dan Shen*), 9g, old Bulbus Allii Fistulosi (*Lao Cong*), 3 stalks, Secretion Moschi Moschiferi (*She Xiang*), 0.3g, Herba Sargassii (*Hai Zao*), 9g, Thallus Algae (*Kun Bu*), 9g, Fructus Zizyphi Jujubae (*Hong Zao*), 5 pieces

E. Central qi insufficiency

Main symptoms: First there is tinnitus; then deafness occurs. The complexion is a sallow yellow. There is fatigue, lack of strength, spiritual fatigue, scant appetite, loose stools, a fine, weak pulse, and a pale tongue with indentations of the teeth on its sides

Treatment principles: Supplement the center and boost the qi, quicken the blood and open the portals

Rx: Radix Astragali Membranacei (*Huang Qi*), 15g, Radix Codonopsis Pilosulae (*Dang Shen*), 10g, Rhizoma Cimicifugae (*Sheng Ma*), 9g, Radix Puerariae (*Ge Gen*), 9g, Fructus Viticis (*Man Jing Zi*), 9g, Radix Dioscoreae Oppositae (*Shan Yao*), 9g, Semen Cuscutae (*Tu Si Zi*), 9g, Cortex Eucommiae Ulmoidis (*Du Zhong*), 9g, Radix Ligustici Wallichii (*Chuan Xiong*), 9g, Rhizoma Acori Graminei (*Chang Pu*), 9g

F. Essence blood deficiency detriment

Main symptoms: Tinnitus, deafness, dizziness and vertigo, lusterless lips and nails, chilled limbs, low back soreness, impotence, premature ejaculation, a fine pulse, and a pale but darkish tongue

Treatment principles: Supplement and boost the liver and kidneys, quicken the blood and open the portals

Rx: Semen Cuscutae (*Tu Si Zi*), 9g, Herba Cistanchis (*Cong Rong*), 9g, Radix Morindae Officinalis (*Ba Ji Tian*), 9g, Radix Angelicae Sinensis (*Dang Gui*), 9g, Cornu Cervi (*Lu Jiao Pian*), 9g, mix-fried Plastrum Testudinis (*Gui Ban*), 9g, Fructus Lycii Chinensis (*Gou Qi Zi*), 9g, Radix Rubrus Paeoniae Lactiflorae (*Chi Shao*), 9g, Radix Ligustici Wallichii (*Chuan Xiong*), 9g, Rhizoma Acori Graminei (*Chang Pu*), 9g, Radix Clematidis Chinensis (*Wei Ling Xian*), 9g, Flos Carthami Tinctorii (*Hong Hua*), 9g

Secret essentials

1. If this pathocondition occurs suddenly, it may be cured rather easily. However, it is difficult to treat this condition if it has endured for many days since it is due to liver/kidney dual deficiency. I use the methods of attacking and supplementing simultaneously, employing Wang Qing-ren's *Tong Qi San* (Open the Qi Powder): Radix Bupleuri (*Chai Hu*), 30g, Rhizoma Cyperi Rotundi (*Xiang Fu*), 30g, Radix Ligustici Wallichii (*Chuan Xiong*), 5g. These ingredients are mixed together and powdered. The dose is 9g each time taken 1 time in the morning and

evening. This powder is washed down with a decoction of 30g of Radix Astragali Membranacei (*Huang Qi*). This moves the qi and diffuses depression, opens the portals and quickens the blood. It is effective in the treatment of tinnitus and deafness.

2. For enduring disease which have not been cured after prolonged treatment, it is all right to use mix-fried Eupolyphaga Seu Opisthoplatia (*Di Bie*), 5g, Sanguis Draconis (*Xue Jie*), 2.4g, Buthus Martensi (*Quan Xie*), 1.5g, Scolopendra Subspinipes (*Wu Gong*), 2 pieces, Periostracum Cicadae (*Chan Yi*), 6g, Radix Puerariae (*Ge Gen*), 9g, Rhizoma Cimicifugae (*Sheng Ma*), 4.5g, Radix Clematidis Chinensis (*Wei Ling Xian*), 15g. Use 500ml of yellow wine (*i.e.*, rice wine), decoct and administer. This opens the portals and diffuses blockage and has a good short-term therapeutic effect.

8. Vertigo & dizziness (*Xuan Yun*)

Vertigo means confused eyesight, while dizziness means dizziness of the head. These two often appear together and are called collectively vertigo and dizziness. Patients with this pathocondition see things as though they were dark or spinning. They feel as if they were sitting aboard a ship or in a car. This condition is often accompanied by nausea and vomiting. One may even not be able to stand and may fall down in a faint.

Disease causes, disease mechanisms

In the *Nei Jing (Inner Classic)*, there is the saying, "Various winds turn into dizziness; these pertain to the liver." The liver is the viscus of wind wood. In body it is yin, but in function is yang. It rules stirring and it rules upbearing. If true yin is insufficient, liver yang may become hyperactive above. Or if water does not moisten wood, wood will have scant enrichment and construction. All this is able to cause wind yang to harass above. The disease mechanism is that there is exuberance above and vacuity below. If bedroom affairs are undisciplined, kidney essence will become deficient and consumed. The sea of marrow will become empty and vacuous. This is categorized as both upper and lower vacuity. The *Jin Gui Yao Lue (Essentials from the Golden Cabinet)* says, "If below the heart there is phlegm rheum, the chest and lateral costal regions will feel full and their will be vertigo." This is because the spleen and stomach transportation and transformation have lost their normalcy. Dampness gathers and becomes phlegm. This then obstructs the clear yang qi. This pattern is characterized by vertigo without dizziness. This is what Zhu Dan-xi meant by saying, "Without phlegm, there is no vertigo." However, I think that static blood may obstruct the channels and vessels. In that case, it is often seen that qi and blood cannot construct and nourish the head and eyes. The ancients did not elaborate on this point.

Treatment based on pattern discrimination

A. Liver yang hyperactive above

Main symptoms: Vertigo, dizziness, tinnitus, headache, head distention occurring during vexation, fatigue, or anger, a bitter taste in the mouth, scanty sleep, a wiry pulse, and a red tongue with yellow coating

Treatment principles: Subdue yang and search wind, level the liver and transform stasis

Rx: Goat Horn (*Shan Yang Jiao*), 30g, Concha Haliotidis (*Shi Jue Ming*), 30g, Radix Salviae Miltiorrhizae (*Dan Shen*), 9g, Radix Scrophulariae Ningpoensis (*Xuan Shen*), 9g, Fructus Gardeniae Jasminoidis (*Shan Zhi*), 9g, Radix Scutellariae Baicalensis (*Huang Qin*), 9g, Ramulus Uncariae Cum Uncis (*Gou Teng*), 15g, Rhizoma Gastrodiae Elatae (*Tian Ma*), 9g, Radix Achyranthis Bidentatae (*Niu Xi*), 9g, Herba Leonuri Heterophylli (*Yi Mu Cao*), 9g, Medulla Tetrapanacis Papyriferi (*Tong Tian Cao*), 9g

B. Kidney essence insufficiency

Main Symptoms: Vertigo, dizziness, weak constitution, essence spirit withering and wilting, a lusterless complexion, low back and knee soreness and weakness, loss of auditory acuity in both ears, a fine pulse, and a pale tongue

Treatment principles: Supplement and boost kidney essence, quicken the blood and nourish the marrow

Rx: Prepared Radix Rehmanniae (*Shu Di*), 15g, Plastrum Testudinis (*Gui Ban*), 15g, Cortex Eucommiae Ulmoidis (*Du Zhong*), 9g, Fructus Lycii Chinensis (*Gou Qi Zi*), 9g, Radix Angelicae Sinensis (*Dang Gui*), 9g, Semen Cuscutae (*Tu Si Zi*), 9g, Radix Achyranthis Bidentatae (*Niu Xi*), 9g, Sclerotium Poriae Cocos (*Fu Ling*), 9g, Cornu Degelatinum Cervi (*Lu Jiao Shuang*), 9g, Semen Pruni Persicae (*Tao Ren*), 9g, *Ci Zhu Wan* (Magnetite & Cinnabar Pills), 9g, Medulla Tetrapanacis Papyriferi (*Tong Tian Cao*), 9g

C. Phlegm turbidity obstructing the center

Main symptoms: Vertigo, a heavy head as if covered, chest oppression, nausea, scanty appetite, excessive sleep, a white, slimy tongue coating, and a soggy, slippery pulse

Treatment principles: Dry dampness and fortify the spleen, eliminate phlegm and transform stasis

Rx: Rhizoma Pinelliae Ternatae (*Ban Xia*), 9g, Rhizoma Atractylodis (*Cang Zhu*), 9g, Rhizoma Atractylodis Macrocephalae (*Bai Zhu*), 9g, Rhizoma Cimicifugae (*Sheng Ma*), 9g, Folium Nelumbinis Nuciferae (*He Ye*), 9g, Rhizoma Gastrodiae Elatae (*Tian Ma*), 9g, Rhizoma Alismatis (*Ze Xie*), 9g, Exocarpium Citri Rubri (*Ju Hong*), 6g, Sclerotium Poriae Cocos (*Fu Ling*), 9g, Fructus Immaturus Citri Seu Ponciri (*Zhi Shi*), 9g, ginger(-processed) Caulis In Taeniis Bambusae (*Zhu Ru*),

6g, Semen Pruni Persicae (*Tao Ren*), 9g, Medulla Tetrapanacis Papyriferi (*Tong Tian Cao*), 9g

D. Stasis obstructing the channels & vessels

Main symptoms: Vertigo and dizziness, headache, head distention, poor memory, loss of sleep, vexation and agitation, easy anger, a purple tongue with static patches, and a wiry, choppy pulse

Treatment principles: Move the blood and open the network vessels, eliminate phlegm, and engender the new

Rx: Radix Angelicae Sinensis (*Dang Gui*), 9g, Radix Rubrus Paeoniae Lactiflorae (*Chi Shao*), 9g, Semen Pruni Persicae (*Tao Ren*), 9g, Flos Carthami Tinctorii (*Hong Hua*), 9g, uncooked Pollen Typhae (*Pu Huang*), 9g, wrapped during decoction, Medulla Tetrapanacis Papyriferi (*Tong Tian Cao*), 9g, Radix Ligustici Wallichii (*Chuan Xiong*), 9g, uncooked Radix Rehmanniae (*Sheng Di*), 9g, Radix Achyranthis Bidentatae (*Niu Xi*), 9g, Radix Platycodi Grandiflori (*Jie Geng*), 4.5g, Radix Bupleuri (*Chai Hu*), 4.5g, Radix Glycyrrhizae (*Gan Cao*), 3g, Fructus Citri Seu Ponciri (*Zhi Qiao*), 4.5g

Secret essentials

1. Although the causes of this disease are phlegm, fire, wind, and vacuity, yet they are all related to static blood. The elderlys' liver and kidneys are insufficient. Water thus fails to irrigate wood. Wind yang ascends and takes advantage. Liver wind comes with phlegm. This is often the precursor of wind stroke. However, in the final analysis, there is still blood stasis in the vessels and network vessels. Thus clear yang suffers being covered. Therefore, I usually use medicinals which quicken the blood and transform stasis to achieve the therapeutic effect. Based on pattern discrimination, medicinals are added to the above formulas to eliminate stasis and open the network vessels. This is really

a great advance in recent years in the treatment principles of TCM.

2. Whenever diseases of the clear portals are treated, it is appropriate to add a little of such medicinals as Herba Menthae Haplocalycis (*Bo He*), Periostracum Cicadae (*Chan Yi*), and Medulla Tetrapanacis Papyriferi (*Tong Tian Cao*). These not only course and scatter wind heat, sweep away phlegm and clear the portals but also work wonders in conducting the channels.

3. During ordinary times (*i.e.*, when the patient is not experiencing dizziness and vertigo), *Heng Fa Sheng Fang* (Balancing Method Sagelike Formula) is administered, 1 packet each time, 2 times per day. This can both treat and prevent various types of vertigo and dizziness.

9. Headache (*Tou Tong*)

Headache is one of the so-called miscellaneous diseases. It may appear due either to external invasion or internal damage. It is a commonly seen pathocondition in clinical practice, and sometimes it may even be the patient's major complaint. According to the *Nei Jing (Inner Classic)*, headache may proceed from the six channels. Headache categorized as *tai yang* proceeds from the posterior part of the head and ascends to the vertex. The pain extends to the nape of the neck and the upper back. If it is categorized as *yang ming*, the pain is in the forehead and involves the eyeballs. If it is categorized as *shao yang*, it reaches the two corners of the head. If it is categorized as *jue yin*, the pain is at the vertex and vomiting of frothy drool occurs. Although the two channels of the *tai yin* and *shao yin* do not reach the head, if phlegm qi counterflows and congests in the diaphragm, clear qi will not be able to reach the head. Therefore, headache and dizziness may often be seen. Thus pattern discrimination based on channel differentiation plays a guiding role in selecting formulas and using medicinals in the treatment of headache.

Disease causes, disease mechanisms

The head is the gathering of all yang. The essence flourishing of the five viscera and the qi of clear yang all concentrate there. If one lives without caution, sits or lies down in the wind, suffers cold, or is rashly exposed to summerheat, then external evils and the six environmental excesses may invade the three yang channels. When such invasion reaches the head, it causes headache. If the disease is enduring and is not cured, phlegm stasis will obstruct and join in the network vessel pathways. Thus head wind disease occurs. Further, if one's emotions and orientation are not harmonious, the liver may lose its coursing and discharging. Depression may then transform into fire, harassing above the clear portals. Headache may also be due to kidney water insufficiency. In that case, water may fail to irrigate wood. Liver yang may then become hyperactive above. If one's natural endowment is not replete, essence and blood may not be able to construct and nourish, or if there is internal damage and stasis obstruction, clear yang may not obtain its proper unfolding and spread. It is also possible that, if one takes too much sweet, fatty food, phlegm dampness may be internally engendered, congesting and holding back the qi mechanism. All these are capable of resulting in the onset of headache.

Treatment based on pattern discrimination

A. Wind cold headache

Main symptoms: Headache radiating to the nape of the neck and upper back, fear of wind and aversion to cold, pain exacerbated by exposure to wind and cold, fondness for covering one's head with a scarf, a pale, white tongue coating, and a floating, tight pulse

Treatment principles: Course wind and scatter cold, quicken the blood and open the network vessels

Rx: Radix Ligustici Wallichii (*Chuan Xiong*), 15g, Radix Angelicae Dahuricae (*Bai Zhi*), 9g, Radix Et Rhizoma Notopterygii (*Qiang Huo*), 9g, Radix Ledebouriellae Sesloidis (*Fang Feng*), 9g, Fructus Viticis (*Man Jing Zi*), 9g, Buthus Martensi (*Quan Xie*), 1.5g, Scolopendra Subspinipes (*Wu Gong*), 2 pieces, Flos Carthami Tinctorii (*Hong Hua*), 9g, Semen Pruni Persicae (*Tao Ren*), 9g, Radix Rubrus Paeoniae Lactiflorae (*Chi Shao*), 9g, Folium Cassiae Occidentalis (*Wang Jiang Nan*), 9g, Folium Photiniae (*Shi Nan Ye*), 9g

B. Liver yang headache

Main symptoms: Headache, heart vexation, easy anger, insomnia, red, hot face, dry throat and mouth, red eyes, a bitter taste in the mouth, constipation and urinary retention, a thin, yellow tongue coating, and a wiry, rapid pulse

Treatment principles: Level the liver and subdue yang, quicken the blood and transform stasis

Rx: Rhizoma Gastrodiae Elatae (*Tian Ma*), 4.5g, Ramulus Uncariae Cum Uncis (*Gou Teng*), 15g, Goat Horn (*Shan Yang Jiao*), 30g, Radix Ligustici Wallichii (*Chuan Xiong*), 15g, Flos Chrysanthemi Morifolii (*Ju Hua*), 9g, Semen Cassiae Torae (*Jue Ming Zi*), 30g, Radix Scutellariae Baicalensis (*Huang Qin*), 9g, Sichuan Rhizoma Coptidis Chinensis (*Chuan Lian*), 2.4g, Cortex Radicis Moutan (*Dan Pi*), 9g, Radix Rubrus Paeoniae Lactiflorae (*Chi Shao*), 9g, Buthus Martensi (*Quan Xie*), 1.5g, Radix Gentianae Scabrae (*Long Dan Cao*), 9g, Radix Et Rhizoma Rhei (*Da Huang*), 9g

C. Blood vacuity headache

Main symptoms: Headache, dizziness, a lusterless complexion, heart palpitations, racing heart, spiritual fatigue, lack of strength, a pale tongue, and a vacuous, fine, choppy pulse

Treatment principles: Enrich and supplement yin, quicken and nourish the blood

Rx: Prepared Radix Rehmanniae (*Shu Di*), 15g, Radix Rubrus Paeoniae Lactiflorae (*Chi Shao*), 9g, Radix Ligustici Wallichii (*Chuan Xiong*), 9g, Radix Angelicae Sinensis (*Dang Shen*), 9g, Radix Salviae Miltior-rhizae (*Dan Shen*), 15g, processed Radix Polygoni Multiflori (*Shou Wu*), 9g, Fructus Tribuli Terrestris (*Bai Ji Li*), 9g, Rhizoma Gastrodiae Elatae (*Tian Ma*), 4.5g, Flos Chrysanthemi Morifolii (*Ju Hua*), 9g, Fructus Lycii Chinensis (*Qi Zi*), 9g, Fructus Ligustri Lucidi (*Nu Zhen Zi*), 9g, Semen Glycinis Hispidae (*Hei Dou*), 9g

D. Static blood headache

Main symptoms: Persistent headache without cure, a dark, stagnant complexion, pain fixed in a certain spot, pain like being pierced by an awl, typically a history of external injury to the head, a purple tongue with static patches, and a choppy pulse

Treatment principles: Quicken the blood and transform stasis, open the network vessels and stop pain

Rx: Radix Bupleuri (*Chai Hu*), 9g, Flos Carthami Tinctorii (*Hong Hua*), 9g, Radix Ligustici Wallichii (*Chuan Xiong*), 15g, Semen Pruni Persicae (*Tao Ren*), 9g, Radix Rubrus Paeoniae Lactiflorae (*Chi Shao*), 9g, Radix Achyranthis Bidentatae (*Niu Xi*), 9g, uncooked Radix Rehmanniae (*Sheng Di*), 9g, Radix Glycyrrhizae (*Gan Cao*), 3g, Fructus Citri Seu Ponciri (*Zhi Qiao*), 4.5g, Radix Platycodi Grandiflori (*Jie Geng*), 4.5g, Radix Angelicae Sinensis (*Dang Gui*), 9g, Nidus Vespae (*Feng Fang*), 9g

Secret essentials

1. One should select different medicinals to conduct the channels based on the region of the head that is painful and channels and network

vessel theory. This helps manifest the full effects of the medicinals used. For instance, in the case of *tai yang* headache, Notopterygium and Vitex should be added. For *yang ming* headache, add Pueraria and Angelica Dahurica. For *shao yang* headache, add Bupleurum and Ligusticum Wallichium. For *jue yin* headache, add Fructus Evodiae Rutecarpae (*Wu Zhu Yu*) and Radix Et Rhizoma Ligustici Chinensis (*Gao Ben*). For *shao yin* headache, add Herba Cum Radice Asari Seiboldi (*Xi Xin*), and, in the case of *tai yin* headache, add Rhizoma Cimicifugae (*Sheng Ma*).

2. For obstinate headaches, I use *Tao Hong Si Wu Tang* (Persica & Carthamus Four Materials Decoction): Semen Pruni Persicae (*Tao Ren*), Flos Carthami Tinctorii (*Hong Hua*), Radix Rubrus Paeoniae Lactiflorae (*Chi Shao*), Radix Angelicae Sinensis (*Dang Gui*), Radix Ligustici Wallichii (*Chuan Xiong*), uncooked Radix Rehmanniae (*Sheng Di*). The weight of Ligusticum may be increased to 30g, and, in addition, 9g of Notopterygium may be added for more satisfactory effect.

3. Taking only two medicinals, *i.e.*, equal amounts of powdered Buthus Martensi (*Quan Xie*) and powdered Scoplopendra Subspinipes (*Wu Gong*), 1.5g each time, 2 times per day, may provide immediate relief.

4. Nine grams of Folium Photiniae (*Shi Nan Ye*) and Folium Cassiae Occidentalis (*Wang Jiang Nan*) should be added to the above formulas in order to raise their therapeutic effect.

10. Insomnia (*Bu Mian*)

Insomnia is also called loss of sleep. The clinical manifestations of this disease are not all the same. Some people cannot sleep when they first go to bed. Others may sleep well at first but awake at midnight. Still others are easily roused from sleep which is interrupted now and then. Some are as if in a trance when they fall asleep but then are frequently startled out of their sleep. Others are not sound asleep but have many fantastic dreams. They roll about restlessly and cannot sleep all night.

Disease causes, disease mechanisms

Static blood may obstruct the chest internally, thus inhibiting the hundreds of vessels. Hence defensive qi may not be able enter and join with the yin aspect. Therefore, sleep is not peaceful or, even during sleep, one may not always close their eyes. One may also have taxation fatigue due to excessive thinking and worry. In that case, the spirit may not keep its place and hence there are heart palpitations and insomnia. If yin is deficient and fire is effulgent, solitary yang may float about. The spirit does not remain quiet at its original place. Thus heart vexation and insomnia occur. Or the heart and gallbladder qi may be driven away. In that case, one is easily frightened and their sleep is harassed by many dreams. There is vacuity vexation and insomnia. Also, if one's eating and drinking are undisciplined, the stomach qi may lose its harmony. It is said, "If the stomach is not harmonious, one cannot lie down quietly."

Treatment based on pattern discrimination

A. Stasis in the blood mansion

Main symptoms: Insomnia, inability for anything to be on one's chest when they lie down at night, the ability to enter sleep only if one takes repressing formulas, chest pain, daybreak perspiration, oppression and vexatious heat within the heart, heart (*i.e.*, mind) busy, heart skipping, lack of tranquility, a purple tongue, and a wiry pulse

Treatment principles: Quicken the blood and transform stasis, course and disinhibit the hundreds of vessels

Rx: Uncooked Radix Rehmanniae (*Sheng Di*), 9g, Radix Angelicae

Sinensis (*Dang Gui*), 9g, Radix Rubrus Paeoniae Lactiflorae (*Chi Shao*), 9g, Radix Ligustici Wallichii (*Chuan Xiong*), 6g, Flos Carthami Tinctorii (*Hong Hua*), 9g, Semen Pruni Persicae (*Tao Ren*), 9g, Radix Bupleuri (*Chai Hu*), 4.5g, Radix Platycodi Grandiflori (*Jie Geng*), 4.5g, Fructus Citri Seu Ponciri (*Zhi Qiao*), 4.5g, Radix Achyranthis Bidentatae (*Niu Xi*), 6g, Radix Glycyrrhizae (*Gan Cao*), 3g

B. Heart/spleen insufficiency

Main symptoms: Excessive dreams, easily awoken, heart palpitations, poor memory, spiritual fatigue, lack of strength, devitalized appetite, scant luster to the facial complexion, a pale tongue with thin coating, and a fine, weak pulse

Treatment principles: Supplement and nourish the heart and spleen, boost the qi and quicken the blood

Rx: Radix Codonopsis Pilosulae (*Dang Shen*), 9g, Rhizoma Atractylodis Macrocephalae (*Bai Zhu*), 9g, Sclerotium Poriae Cocos (*Fu Ling*), 9g, stir-fried Semen Ziziphi Spinosae (*Zao Ren*), 9g, Radix Astragali Membranacei (*Huang Qi*), 15g, Radix Angelicae Sinensis (*Dang Shen*), 9g, Radix Saussureae Seu Vladimiriae (*Mu Xiang*), 3g, mix-fried Radix Glycyrrhizae (*Zhi Gan Cao*), 3g, Radix Ligustici Wallichii (*Chuan Xiong*), 4.5g, Radix Polygalae Tenuifoliae (*Yuan Zhi*), 9g, Fructus Schizandrae Chinensis (*Wu Wei Zi*), 6g, Pinellia Massa Medica Fermentata (*Ban Xia Qu*), 9g, Semen Biotae Orientalis (*Bai Zi Ren*), 9g, Radix Salviae Miltiorrhizae (*Dan Shen*), 10g, Arillus Euphoriae Longanae (*Long Yan Rou*), 7 pieces

C. Yin deficiency, fire effulgence

Main symptoms: Heart vexation, insomnia, dizziness, vertigo, tinnitus, spermatorrhea, premature ejaculation, vexatious heat in the five hearts, heart palpitations, easy fright, a red tongue, and a fine, rapid pulse

Treatment principles: Enrich yin and downbear fire, clear the heart and transform stasis

Rx: Radix Scrophulariae Ningpoensis (*Xuan Shen*), 9g, Radix Salviae Miltiorrhizae (*Dan Shen*), 15g, Tuber Asparagi Cochinensis (*Tian Dong*), 9g, Cortex Phellodendri (*Huang Bai*), 9g, uncooked Radix Rehmanniae (*Sheng Di*), 12g, Radix Glycyrrhizae (*Gan Cao*), 3g, Fructus Amomi (*Sha Ren*), 2.4g, Sclerotium Pararadicis Poriae Cocos (*Fu Shen*), 9g, Radix Rubrus Paeoniae Lactiflorae (*Chi Shao*), 9g, Radix Angelicae Sinensis (*Dang Gui*), 9g, Succinum (*Hu Bo*), 1.5g, added after the other ingredients are decocted

D. Heart/gallbladder qi timidity

Main symptoms: Heart palpitations, excessive dreams, easy fright, sleep not quiet, a pale tongue with thin coating, and a fine, slippery pulse

Treatment principles: Boost the qi and settle fright, quicken the blood and quiet the spirit

Rx: Uncooked and prepared Semen Ziziphi Spinosae (*Zao Ren*), 9g @, Sclerotium Poriae Cocos (*Fu Ling*), 9g, Radix Ligustici Wallichii (*Chuan Xiong*), 9g, Rhizoma Anemarrhenae (*Zhi Mu*), 9g, Radix Glycyrrhizae (*Gan Cao*), 3g, Radix Polygalae Tenuifoliae (*Yuan Zhi*), 9g, Rhizoma Acori Graminei (*Chang Pu*), 9g, Os Draconis (*Long Gu*), 30g, Plastrum Testudinis (*Gui Ban*), 15g, prepared Radix Rehmanniae (*Shu Di*), 15g, Fructus Alpiniae Oxyphyllae (*Yi Zhi Ren*), 9g

E. Stomach center disharmony

Main symptoms: Loss of sleep, epigastric oppression, distention, and fullness, belching, abdominal discomfort, inhibited defecation, a yellow, slimy tongue coating, and a slippery, rapid pulse

Treatment principles: Harmonize the stomach and transform accumulations, disperse and conduct stasis heat

Rx: Rhizoma Coptidis Chinensis (*Huang Lian*), 3g, Fructus Gardeniae Jasminoidis (*Shan Zhi*), 9g, Fructus Immaturus Citri Seu Ponciri (*Zhi Shi*), 9g, Radix Platycodi Grandiflori (*Jie Geng*), 6g, Rhizoma Pinelliae Ternatae (*Ban Xia*), 9g, Northern Sanon Petarie Italicae   (*Shu Mi*), 9g, wrapped during decoction, Massa Medica Fermentata (*Shen Qu*), 9g, Radix Salviae Miltiorrhizae (*Dan Shen*), 15g, Cortex Albizziae Julibrissinis (*He Huan Pi*), 9g, Caulis in Taeniis Bambusae (*Zhu Ru*), 6g

Secret essentials

1. Insomnia also encompasses the phenomenon where, as soon as one closes their eyes, they have dreams in which they see strange or weird figures. It may also refer to being startled by nightmare with loud shrieks. during the day, there is chest and lateral costal bitterness (*i.e.*, Pain) and fullness. After noon there is an abnormal feeling of heat. Now and then, one may weep. Their complexion is dark and blackish. The pulse is wiry and the surface of the tongue has purple qi (*i.e.*, is purplish in color). Ordinary people do not know this strange disease. Therefore, it is ineffective to consult the doctors. For this, I administer *Xue Fu Zhu Yu Tang* (Blood Mansion Dispel Stasis Decoction) accompanied by 1.5g of Succinum (*Hu Bo*) and 9g of Rhizoma Acori Graminei (*Chan Pu*). Every shot necessarily hits the mark.

2. The elderly do not sleep well at night, while in broad daylight, they become drowsy and desire sleep. The *Nei Jing (Inner Classic)* states:

> Constructive and defensive normally construct the corporeal and ethereal souls. If the spirit is over-taxed, the corporeal and ethereal souls will scatter. Then the orientation will become chaotic.

In order to nourish the spirit, first treat the qi and blood, regulate and contain the constructive and defensive, and balance yin and yang by regularly taking *Heng Fa Sheng Fang* (Balancing Method Sagelike Formula) and one will get the effect.

3. Old peoples' qi and blood is debilitated and astringent. Therefore, one should make scant use of medicinals which supplement yang and strengthen yang. In the *Nei Jing (Inner Classic)*, there is the wise precept:

> If yang qi is exuberant, the eyes will stare. If yin qi is exuberant, the eyes will close.

The Chinese ready-made medicine *Tian Wang Bu Xin Dan* (Heavenly Emperor Supplement the Heart Elixir) is quite suitable for the body, *i.e.*, constitution, of the elderly. If one adds 0.3g of powdered Rhizoma Coptidis Chinensis (*Huang Lian*) to various formulas for insomnia and washes this down with the decoction before going to bed, then one will get a prompt effect.

11. Heart palpitations (*Xin Ji*) & racing heart (*Zheng Chong*)

Heart palpitations occur when, without fright, one feels that their heart throbs uncomfortably, spasmodically, and uncontrollably. Racing heart is when the heart skips and there is lack of tranquility. The heart goes thump-thump and the spirit shakes. Heart racing is more serious than heart palpitations. Heart palpitations may be divided into vacuity or repletion, while heart racing is mostly categorized as a vacuity pattern.

Disease causes, disease mechanisms

If heart qi is insufficient, it is not able to transport and propel blood flow normally. If heart blood is deficient internally, it is not able to construct and nourish the vessels and pathways, making them full, exuberant, regulated, and coursing. The heart thus loses its nourishment, and the spirit is not tranquil but abandons its place. Hence, there is often the signs of heart fluster and timidity. If the disease endures and is not cured, then the heart becomes vexed and chaotic, lying down is not quiet, and sleep is harassed by dreams. Food and drink have scant flavor. This may also be caused by heart yang being devitalized. In that case, there is recurrent invasion by external evils. All these are mutually related to static blood.

Treatment based on pattern discrimination

A. Heart loss of nourishment

Main symptoms: Heart palpitations, restlessness, sleep at night not tranquil, a lusterless complexion, in severe cases, racing heart with perspiration, tinnitus, and blurred vision, a pale red tongue with a thin, white coating, and a fine, weak pulse

Treatment principles: Boost the qi and quicken the blood, nourish the blood and quiet the spirit

Rx: Radix Codonopsis Pilosulae (*Dang Shen*), 9g, Tuber Ophiopogonis Japonicae (*Mai Dong*), 9g, Fructus Schizandrae Chinensis (*Wu Wei Zi*), 6g, Sclerotium Pararadicis Poriae Cocos (*Fu Shen*), 9g, prepared Radix Rehmanniae (*Shu Di*), 15g, Radix Angelicae Sinensis (*Dang Gui*), 9g, Radix Ligustici Wallichii (*Chuan Xiong*), 6g, Radix Glycyrrhizae (*Gan Cao*), 3g, uncooked and prepared Semen Ziziphi Spinosae (*Zao Ren*), 9g @, Semen Biotae Orientalis (*Bai Zi Ren*), 9g, Os Draconis (*Long Gu*), 30g, Fructus Alpiniae Oxyphyllae (*Yi Zhi Ren*), 9g, Radix Salviae Miltiorrhizae (*Dan Shen*), 15g

B. Stasis in the blood mansion

Main symptoms: Heart palpitations, susceptibility to fright, easy fear, racing heart, scant sleep, chest oppression, lateral costal fullness, internal vexation, an abnormal feeling of heat, tenseness, agitation, excessive anger, a dark red tongue, distended, engorged, greenish blue sinews under the tongue, and a wiry, choppy pulse

Treatment principles: Settle the spirit and tranquilize the ethereal soul, quicken the blood and transform stasis

Rx: Semen Pruni Persicae (*Tao Ren*), 9g, Flos Carthami Tinctorii (*Hong Hua*), 9g, Radix Salviae Miltiorrhizae (*Dan Shen*), 15g, Radix Angelicae Sinensis (*Dang Gui*), 9g, Os Draconis (*Long Gu*), 30g, Concha Ostreae (*Mu Li*), 30g, Ramulus Cinnamomi (*Gui Zhi*), 6g, Radix Rubrus Paeoniae Lactiflorae (*Chi Shao*), 9g, Radix Albus Paeoniae Lactiflorae (*Bai Shao*), 9g, mix-fried Radix Glycyrrhizae (*Zhi Gan Cao*), 4.5g, Radix Ligustici Wallichii (*Chuan Xiong*), 9g, Tuber Curcumae (*Yu Jin*), 9g, Resina Olibani (*Ru Xiang*), 4.5g, Magnetitum (*Ci Shi*), 30g

Secret essentials

1. If one feels their heart beating irregularly due to external unfavorable stimulation, that is called fright. If there is no fright but the heart throbs uncomfortably, this is called palpitation. If, out of one's control, the heart throbs and skips, this known as racing heart. Generally, whenever something provokes sudden fear, qi and blood suddenly gather. After a while, the patient will feel somewhat relieved. If they toss about in bed and worry about things, qi and blood will congeal and collect. Thus stasis will be retained in the blood mansion. It is usually of no avail if one begins simply by nourishing the blood and quieting the spirit. However, if medicinals are added to harmonize and quicken the blood, transform stasis and open the network vessels, then the situation can be suddenly changed for the better.

2. The pattern of internal timidity is related to one's emotions and orientation. This primarily arises due to qi chaos and blood stasis. If *Xue*

Fu Zhu Yu Tang (Blood Mansion Dispel Stasis Decoction) is administered, there are usually good results. (The ingredients of this formula are given in the section on impotence.) If the disease endures without being cured, one may administer mix-fried Radix Glycyrrhizae (*Zhi Gan Cao*), 6g, Fructus Levis Tritici (*Huai Xiao Mai*), 15g, Fructus Zizyphi Jujubae (*Da Zao*), 5 pieces, calcined Os Draconis (*Long Gu*) and Concha Ostreae (*Mu Li*), 15g @, Radix Salviae Miltiorrhizae (*Dan Shen*), 9g, Succinum (*Hu Bo*), 1.5g, added after the other ingredients are decocted, with mostly good result.

12. Vacuity taxation (*Xu Lao*)

This pathocondition is also known as vacuity detriment. It is a general term for chronic vacuity and debility diseases with deficiency detriment of the viscera and bowel original qi and essence blood insufficiency as the main pathological changes. Generally, vacuity occurs when the body is feeble after enduring disease. If vacuity endures, it is called detriment. If detriment is carried to extreme, it is called taxation. These three are formed by gradual accumulation.

Disease causes, disease mechanisms

This pathocondition may be caused by external damage, drinking and diet, taxation and fatigue, and by internal damage by the seven emotions and six desires. Over-taxation damages the lungs, melting and smelting lung yin. Sexual desire damages the kidneys, causing the essence chamber to be empty and vacuous. Worry and vain thoughts damage the heart, causing the blood vessels to lose their harmony. Hunger and satiation damage the spleen. Thus the central region does not transport. Anger and jealousy damage the liver. Thus depressive fire blazes recurrently. The Qing Dynasty physician Ma Yuan-yi divided yang vacuity into two and yin vacuity into three. This well explains the problem. The two kinds of yang vacuity are 1) kidney yang vacuity and debility, in which case the former heaven or prenatal natural endowment is already thin;

and 2) spleen/stomach vacuity cold, in which case the latter heaven or postnatal support and protection are incompetent. As to the three kinds of yin vacuity, they are 1) consumption and damage of lung and stomach yin fluids, 2) heart/spleen yin blood vacuity and deficiency, and 3) liver/kidney yin essence deficiency. However, clinically, pure deficiency is seldom observed. In most patterns, vacuity and repletion come together. One of the causes of this is static blood. Retention of stasis is usually the reason why righteous qi is not able to extend and grow and why fresh blood is not engendered once again.

Treatment based on pattern discrimination

A. Kidney yang vacuity & debility

Main symptoms: Low back chill, impotence, premature ejaculation, vertigo and dizziness, a somber, dark complexion, devitalized essence spirit, listlessness, lack of strength, a pale, fat tongue, and deep, slow pulse

Treatment principles: Warm and supplement kidney yang, boost the qi and quicken the blood

Rx: Cornu Cervi (*Lu Jiao Pain*), 9g, Semen Cuscutae (*Tu Si Zi*), 9g, Herba Cistanchis (*Cong Rong*), 9g, Radix Angelicae Sinensis (*Dang Gui*), 9g, Fructus Lycii Chinensis (*Qi Zi*), 9g, Semen Biotae Orientalis (*Bai Zi Ren*), 9g, Fructus Corni Officinalis (*Yu Rou*), 9g, Flos Carthami Tinctorii (*Hong Hua*), 9g, Semen Trigonellae Foeni-graeci (*Hu Lu Ba*), 9g, Fructus Foeniculi Vulgaris (*Xiao Hui Xiang*), 2.4g

B. Spleen/stomach vacuity cold

Main symptoms: Scanty appetite, loose stools, abdominal pain, tenesmus, fear of cold, chilled limbs, a sallow yellow complexion, a pale tongue with white coating, and a vacuous, soft pulse

Treatment principles: Warm the center and fortify the spleen, quicken the blood and supplement the constructive

Rx: Ramulus Cinnamomi (*Gui Zhi*), 6g, Radix Albus Paeoniæ Lactiflorae (*Bai Shao*), 9g, mix-fried Radix Glycyrrhizae (*Zhi Gan Cao*), 4.5g, Radix Astragali Membranacei (*Huang Qi*), 15g, Radix Angelicae Sinensis (*Dang Gui*), 9g, Radix Salviae Miltiorrhizae (*Dan Shen*), 15g, Sclerotium Poriae Cocos (*Fu Ling*), 9g, Rhizoma Atractylodis Macrocephalae (*Bai Zhu*), 9g, roasted Rhizoma Zingiberis (*Wei Jiang*), 2 slices, Fructus Zizyphi Jujubae (*Da Zao*), 5 pieces, and Malt Sugar (*Yi Tang*), 9g, added after the other ingredients are decocted

C. Lung/stomach fluid vacuity

Main symptoms: Bloody cough, shortness of breath, distressed rapid dyspneic breathing, dry throat, loss of voice, tidal fever, steaming bones, night sweats, a flushed red complexion, a red tongue with scant fluids, and a fine, rapid pulse

Treatment principles: Moisten the lungs and quiet the network vessels, harmonize the stomach and engender fluids

Rx: Radix Adenophorae Strictae (*Nan Sha Shen*),9g, Radix Glehniae Littoralis (*Bei Sha Shen*), 9g, Tuber Ophiopogonis Japonicae (*Mai Dong*), 9g, Rhizoma Polygonati Odorati (*Yu Zhu*), 9g, Cortex Radicis Mori Albi (*Sang Pi*), 9g, Cortex Radicis Lycii (*Di Gu Pi*), 9g, uncooked Radix Rehmanniae (*Sheng Di*), 9g, Radix Stellariae Dichotomae (*Yin Chai Hu*), 6g, mix-fried Carapax Amydae Sinensis (*Bie Jia*), 9g, Semen Pruni Persicae (*Tao Ren*), 9g, Semen Benincasae Hispidae (*Dong Gua Zi*), 9g, uncooked Semen Coicis Lachryma-jobi (*Mi Ren*), 30g, Rhizoma Phragmitis Communi (*Lu Gen*), 30g, Nodus Nelumbinis Nuciferae (*Ou Jie*), 9g

D. Heart/spleen blood vacuity

Main symptoms: Fright palpitations, racing heart, poor memory, loss of sleep, vexation and agitation, excessive dreams, night sweats, sores on the mouth and tongue, a flushed red complexion, a scarlet red tongue, and a fine, rapid pulse

Treatment principles: Harmonize and delight the heart and spleen, nourish yin and quicken the blood

Rx: Radix Salviae Miltiorrhizae (*Dan Shen*), 15g, Radix Scrophulariae Ningpoensis (*Xuan Shen*), 9g, Tuber Asparagi Cochinensis (*Tian Dong*), 9g, uncooked Radix Rehmanniae (*Sheng Di*), 12g, Rhizoma Anemarrhenae (*Zhi Mu*), 9g, Radix Ligustici Wallichii (*Chuan Xiong*), 6g, Sclerotium Poriae Cocos (*Fu Ling*), 9g, uncooked & prepared Semen Ziziphi Spinosae (*Zao Ren*), 9g @, Rhizoma Coptidis Chinensis (*Huang Lian*), 2.4g, Radix Angelicae Sinensis (*Dang Gui*), 9g, Radix Glycyrrhizae (*Gan Cao*), 3g

E. Liver/kidney essence vacuity

Main symptoms: Low back soreness, spermatorrhea, throat pain, red cheeks, heart vexation, tinnitus, both feet atonic and weak, a red tongue with scant coating, and a fine, rapid pulse

Treatment principles: Enrich and supplement the liver and kidneys, downbear fire and dispel stasis

Rx: Prepared Radix Rehmanniae (*Shu Di*), 15g, Plastrum Testudinis (*Gui Ban*), 9g, Rhizoma Anemarrhenae (*Zhi Mu*), 9g, Cortex Phellodendri (*Huang Bai*), 9g, Cortex Radicis Moutan (*Dan Pi*), 9g, Rhizoma Alismatis (*Ze Xie*), 9g, Radix Dioscoreae Oppositae (*Shan Yao*), 9g, Fructus Corni Officinalis (*Yu Rou*), 9g, Sclerotium Poriae Cocos (*Fu Ling*), 9g, Tuber Asparagi Cochinensis (*Tian Dong*), 9g, Radix Rubrus

Paeoniae Lactiflorae (*Chi Shao*), 9g, Radix Achyranthis Bidentatae (*Niu Xi*), 9g, stir-fried in salt water

F. Blood stasis internally stopped

Main symptoms: Rough skin, in severe cases, scaly nails like fish scales, emaciation, both eyes dark and blackish, a bluish purple tongue, and a fine, choppy pulse

Treatment principles: Quicken the blood and transform stasis, boost the qi and aid transportation

Rx: Rhizoma Atractylodis (*Cang Zhu*), 9g, Rhizoma Atractylodis Macrocephalae (*Bai Zhu*), 9g, uncooked Pollen Typhae (*Pu Huang*), 9g, wrapped during decoction, Radix Astragali Membranacei (*Huang Qi*), 30g, Rhizoma Curcumae Zedoariae (*E Zhu*), 9g, Radix Codonopsis Pilosulae (*Dang Shen*), 10g, Radix Rubrus Paeoniae Lactiflorae (*Chi Shao*), 9g, Hirudo (*Shui Zhi*), 3g, Radix Angelicae Sinensis (*Dang Gui*), 9g, Radix Ligustici Wallichii (*Chuan Xiong*), 9g, prepared Radix Rehmanniae (*Shu Di*), 30g, Semen Pruni Persicae (*Tao Ren*), 9g, Stigma Croci Sativae (*Zang Hong Hua*), 1.5g, steeped

Secret essentials

1. This pathocondition should first be divided according to bodily yin and yang. Spleen yang should be upborne. If it is vacuous, it will fall and drop. If it is moved, discharged, or downborne, then engendering qi will be checked. Kidney yang should be gathered and concentrated. In case of taxation, it will float about. If it is further moved, upborne, or emitted, then true qi will be extinguished. Yin fluids are engendered from qi. It may engender only clear, moist substances. Yin essence is engendered from taste. It can be fulfilled only by enriching, slimy substances. Yin blood is engendered from water and grain. It can be

transformed only by regulating the central region. Thus one may understand the essence of this formula.

2. One should discriminate between upper, middle, and lower patterns. The physician (*i.e.*, Qi Bo) has said:

> Detriment may go from above to below. If it passes beyond the stomach, it cannot be treated. Detriment may come from below to above. If it passes beyond the spleen, it also cannot be treated.

Therefore, in both treatment and prognosis, spleen and stomach qi are important. Once the function of spleen and stomach fails, it is impossible to make up the deficiencies. In most cases, there will occur untreatable conditions. Thus, I like to use Rhizoma Atraclylodis to blaze the trail and run before, based on the theory that, "The stomach likes of supplementation" and "The spleen unites the four viscera."

3. Where the lungs are damaged, supplement the spleen, and if the liver is vacuous, supplement the kidneys. Fostering both the child and mother is the expedient way to treat vacuity taxation. Moreover, the spleen and kidneys are the former and latter heaven sources of transformation. If these two viscera obtain supplementation, all the other viscera obtain boosting.

4. Supporting the righteous and eliminating evils combined with quickening the blood and transforming stasis are the two great methods in treating vacuity taxation. *Shu Yu Wan* (Dioscorea Pills) is a formula for supplementing both the spleen and the kidneys. Sun Si- miao used Gelatinum Cornu Cervi (*Lu Jiao*) in place of Gelatinum Corii Asini (*E Jiao*) and added Radix Scutellariae Baicalensis (*Huang Qin*), thus creating a formula with a new rationale. *Da Huang Zhe Chong Wan* (Rhubarb & Eupolyphaga Pills) treats dry blood internally with new blood not being able to irrigate and pour. It may be used both for attacking stasis and for nourishing the blood. Thus I base my treatment of vacuity taxation and chronic illness on the essential rationale of the

ancient formulas and on the principles of quickening the blood and transforming stasis, boosting the qi and aiding transportation. Clinical surveys prove that this method is quite effective.

13. Bleeding patterns (*Xue Zheng*)

Blood flow may not follow its regular pathways but may flow upward and spill out of the portals of the mouth and nose. It may descend and exit from the two yin (*i.e.*, the anus and genitals), or it may percolate through the muscles and skin. In general, these conditions are called bleeding patterns. Blood and qi mutually engender and mutually function. Qi carries the blood to circulate cyclically through the channels and vessels. It fills and moistens, constructs and nourishes the entire body. If either yin or yang is preponderant over the other, blood in the channels and vessels will spill over and flow out from the region where debility or damage is markedly manifest. The *Nei Jing* states:

> When the yang network vessels are damaged, blood spills over externally. External spillage of blood results in bleeding. When the yin network vessels are damaged, blood spills over internally. When blood spills over internally, there is bleeding behind (*i.e.*, hemafecia).

The ancients have already discussed the relationship between bleeding patterns and stasis. Therefore, in treating bleeding patterns, it is first necessary to eliminate the cause of disease. If the cause of the disease is not eliminated, the blood network vessels will not be quiet. "For bleeding, do not use the stopping method" is an ancient saying. If, whenever bleeding appears, one stops bleeding, one will wrongly leave behind the disease mechanism.

Disease causes, disease mechanisms

The cause of hemorrhage is usually related to qi, fire, and stasis. The *Jing Yue Quan Shu (The Complete Writings of Jing-yue)* states:

Stirring is mostly due to fire. Fire exuberance forces the blood to move recklessly. Detriment is mostly due to qi. If qi is damaged, blood is not contained.

Qi is the commander of the blood. Blood follows the movement of qi. If fire is effulgent and qi counterflows, then blood will spill over. If cold congeals, then qi stagnates and blood becomes static. However, in terms of the clinical manifestations in the elderly, there are numerous cases where stasis heat is deep-lying internally in the constructive aspect or the qi and blood of the viscera and bowels are deficient and debilitated. Thus this condition can be divided into vacuity and repletion. Repletion is mostly caused by heat toxins which fall internally into the constructive blood. Heat leads to stirring of the blood, while scorching damages the network vessels. It is also possible for stomach heat to be hyperactive and exuberant. Powerful heat may flame upward and force the blood to spill over externally. Vacuity is mostly due to spleen/kidney qi vacuity. These then fail to restrain and contain, with the blood thus not abiding in its place. It is also possible for there to be yin vacuity with fire effulgence. Ministerial fire recklessly stirs and fire and heat harass and stir yin blood. Therefore these are not able to remain tranquil within the network vessels and pathways. Whenever blood leaves the channels, it should be considered as blood stasis. If one does not know this, then stopping bleeding alone will definitely result in retention (of static blood) with its negative consequences.

Treatment based on pattern discrimination

A. Qi counterflow damaging the network vessels

Main symptoms: Spasmodic cough, chest and lateral costal radiating pain, red-looking phlegm, a dry mouth, vexatious heat, epistaxis, bleeding gums, epigastric and abdominal glomus and pain, black-colored stools, dizziness, tidal fever, short, red urination, a red tongue, and a wiry, rapid pulse

Treatment principles: Tranquilize the heart and quiet the network vessels, downbear the qi and transform stasis

Rx: Uncooked Radix Rehmanniae (*Sheng Di*), 15g, uncooked Cacumeñ Biotae Orientalis (*Ce Bai Ye*), 15g, uncooked Folium Artemisiae Argyii (*Ai Ye*), 3g, Folium Nelumbinis Nuciferae (*He Ye*), 9g, Radix Scrophulariae Ningpoensis (*Xuan Shen*), 12g, Radix Achyranthis Bidentatae (*Niu Xi*), 9g, Cortex Radicis Moutan (*Dan Pi*), 9g, Fructus Gardeniae Jasminoidis (*Shan Zhi*), 9g, Radix Rubrus Paeoniae Lactiflorae (*Chi Shao*), 9g, uncooked Pollen Typhae (*Pu Huang*), 9g, wrapped during decoction, Lignum Dalbergiae Odoriferae (*Jiang Xiang*), 2.4g, Cornu Bubali (*Shui Niu Jiao*), 30g

B. Heat brewing & forcing the blood

Main symptoms: Dry throat, agitation and vexation, nose heat, bleeding gums, headache, red eyes, hematuria, constipation, oral thirst leading to drinking, vomiting large amounts of blood, epigastric pain and burning heat, stools precipitating fresh red blood, a red face, mouth sores, piercing pain when urinating, a scarlet red tongue, and a flooding, rapid pulse

Treatment principles: Cool the blood and stop bleeding, clear heat and transform stasis

Rx: Cornu Bubali (*Shui Niu Jiao*), 6g, uncooked Radix Rehmanniae (*Sheng Di*), 60g, Cortex Radicis Moutan (*Dan Pi*), 9g, Radix Rubrus Paeoniae Lactiflorae (*Chi Shao*), 15g, uncooked Radix Et Rhizoma Rhei (*Da Huang*), 9g, Radix Scrophulariae Ningpoensis (*Xuan Shen*), 15g, Radix Achyranthis Bidentatae (*Niu Xi*), 9g

C. Vacuity not containing the blood

Main symptoms: A bloodless white complexion, spiritual fatigue, lack of strength, dizziness, darkening of the eyes, tinnitus, heart palpitations, dripping sweat, dark but pale blood, insidious abdominal pain, no thought for food or drink, a pale but dark tongue, and a fine, weak, choppy pulse

Treatment principles: Fortify the spleen and contain the blood, boost the qi and transform stasis

Rx: Radix Astragali Membranacei (*Huang Qi*), 30g, Radix Codonopsis Pilosulae (*Dang Shen*), 15g, Rhizoma Bletillae Striatae (*Bai Ji*), 12g, Fructus Schizandrae Chinensis (*Wu Wei Zi*), 6g, Tuber Ophiopogonis Japonicae (*Mai Dong*), 9g, Radix Rubiae Cordifoliae (*Qian Cao*), 9g, Os Sepiae Seu Sepiellae (*Wu Zei Gu*), 15g, Rhizoma Atractylodis Macrocephalae (*Bai Zhu*), 9g, prepared Radix Rehmanniae (*Da Shu Di*), 30g, Pollen Typhae stir-fried Gelatinum Corii Asini (*E Jiao*), 9g, Radix Boehmeriae (*Zhu Ma Gen*), 30g, *Yun Nan Bai Yao* (Yunnan White Medicine), 1g, taken separately

Secret essentials

1. In the treatment of hemorrhage, the idea already exists in our national medical theory (*i.e.*, TCM) that, "For bleeding, do not use the stopping method." This idea is beneficial when administering medicinals in clinical practice. Owing to static blood internally obstructing, blood movement does not abide in its pathways and thus bleeding occurs. If the blood outside the channels is not eliminated, it will not only prevent the engenderment of new blood but will aggravate the signs of obstruction and stagnation in the channels and network vessels. This then results in hemorrhaging without stop. Clinically, one may see interstitial hemorrhagic diseases and various other large and small

hemorrhagic patterns. If one cools and scatters the blood, after 1 dose, one may know some effect. Two doses and the condition will be over.

2. If static blood is not removed, the blood in the network vessels will not be quiet. If static blood is not removed, new blood will not be engendered. Thus, when treating the blood, first remove stasis. However, in selecting medicinals, one should take their specific natures into account. I use uncooked Pollen Typhae, Radix Pseudoginseng (*San Qi*), stir-fried Red Peony, stir-fried Moutan, and *Yun Nan Bai Yao* (Yunan White Medicine) to stop bleeding without retaining stasis. This is thus an ideal therapy.

3. Based on clinical experience, I treat bleeding patterns by the four methods of downbearing the qi, clearing away heat, boosting the qi, and transforming stasis. According to pattern discrimination, I have used these methods to treat different kinds of bleeding patterns with satisfactory effects.

14. *Bi* patterns (*Bi Zheng*)

Bi patterns refer to diseases of obstruction and blockage of qi and blood by various evils. Due to qi and blood deficiency and vacuity, the interstices may lose their density. Wind, cold, and damp evils may take advantage of this vacuity and invade the muscular exterior and channels and network vessels. Thus the transportation and movement of the qi and blood is inhibited. This leads to aching and pain, heaviness, and inhibition of bending and stretching of the sinews and bones, muscles and flesh, and joints. It may also lead to swelling and distention of the joints. Clinically, this condition is characterized by repeated occurrences and relapses.

Disease causes, disease mechanisms

The onset of this disease is chiefly due to the constructive and defensive not securing. The interstices are sparse (*i.e.* not densely packed) and wide open. Thus external evils take advantage of this and enter the body. After the occurrence of this disease, it is due to qi and blood transportation and movement being inhibited. Thus there is no power to dispel evils to the outside but rather they join ranks with the external evils, causing stasis and obstruction in the channels. These go deep into the joints, sinews, and vessels. Whenever the weather is windy, rainy, or gloomy and wet, yang qi is arrested and checked and the vessels and network vessels are all the more obstructed, closed, and not free-flowing and the symptoms are exacerbated. If wind is preponderant and moves about without a fixed point, this is called moving *bi*. If dampness is preponderant with swelling, distention, and heaviness, it is called fixed *bi*. If cold is preponderant and there is intense pain, it is called painful *bi*. If the body is yin vacuous and internally there is congestive heat, external evils after entering the body may easily transform into heat. This results in joint redness and swelling and is called heat *bi*. If wind, cold, and wetness endure and are not dispelled, depression will transform into fire. This may also turn into heat *bi*. If *bi* patterns last a long time and recur repeatedly, the joints of the bones become stiff and deformed. Bending and stretching is inhibited. This is called recalcitrant *bi*.

Treatment based on pattern discrimination

A. Moving *bi* (wind *bi*)

Main symptoms: Soreness and pain of the limbs, body, and joints. This pain moves around and is not fixed. It mostly manifests in the big joints, such as the wrists, elbows, ankles, and knees. It may inhibit activity. In the initial stage, it may be accompanied with such symptoms as aversion to cold, fear of wind, fever, and sweating. The tongue coating is thin and white. The pulse is floating and relaxed (retarded).

Treatment principles: Dispel wind and quicken the blood, course and open the channels and network vessels

Rx: Radix Et Rhizoma Notopterygii (*Qiang Huo*), 9g, Radix Angelicae Pubescentis (*Du Huo*), 9g, Radix Gentianae Macrophyllae (*Qin Jiao*), 9g, Radix Ledebouriellae Sesloidis (*Fang Feng*), 9g, Ramulus Mori Albi (*Sang Zhi*), 15g, Radix Angelicae Sinensis (*Dang Gui*), 9g, Radix Ligustici Wallichii (*Chuan xiong*), 9g, Herba Erodii Stephanii (*Lao Guan Cao*), 30g, Herba Siegesbeckiae Orientalis (*Xi Xian Cao*), 15g, processed Resina Olibani (*Ru Xiang*), 4.5g, processed Resina Myrrhae (*Mo Yao*), 4.5g, Caulis Piperis (*Hai Feng Teng*), 9g, Cortex Erythrinae (*Hai Tong Pi*), 9g

B. Painful *bi* (cold *bi*)

Main symptoms: Aching and pain of the limbs, body, and joints, light pain in the day, more severe at night, exacerbated by cold but mitigated when it obtains warmth, inhibition in bending and stretching the joints, chilly feeling at the place of pain, a white tongue coating, and a tight or slow pulse

Treatment principles: Warm the channels and scatter cold, quicken the blood and open the network vessels

Rx: Radix Aconiti (*Wu Tou*), 9g, Herba Ephedrae (*Ma Huang*), 9g, Radix Astragali Membranacei (*Huang Qi*), 30g, Radix Albus Paeoniae Lactiflorae (*Bai Shao*), 9g, Radix Glycyrrhizae (*Gan Cao*), 6g, Ramulus Cinnamomi (*Gui Zhi*), 4.5g, Rhizoma Atractylodis (*Cang Zhu*), 9g, wine(-processed) Lumbricus (*Di Long*), 6g, Herba Cum Radice Asari Seiboldi (*Xi Xin*), 4.5g, Rhizoma Arisaematis (*Nan Xing*), 6g, processed

Resina Olibani (*Ru Xiang*), 4.5g, processed Resina Myrrhae (*Mo Yao*), 4.5g, Flos Carthami Tinctorii (*Hong Hua*), 9g

C. Fixed *bi* (damp *bi*)

Main symptoms: Aching and pain of the limbs, body, joints, muscles, and flesh which is fixed at a certain spot and has a markedly heavy or numb sensation, swelling and distention of the affected area, activity not quick, a pale tongue with a white, slimy coating, and a soggy, relaxed (retarded) pulse

Treatment principles: Open the channels and dispel dampness, quicken the blood and transform stasis

Rx: Rhizoma Atractylodis (*Cang Zhu*), 9g, Radix Stephaniae Tetrandrae (*Fang Ji*), 9g, Semen Coicis Lachryma-jobi (*Yi Ren*), 30g, Herba Ephedrae (*Ma Huang*), 9g, Semen Pruni Armeniacae (*Xing Ren*), 9g, Ramulus Cinnamomi (*Gui Zhi*), 6g, Radix Glycyrrhizae (*Gan Cao*), 3g, Radix Angelicae Sinensis (*Dang Gui*), 9g, Radix Ligustici Wallichii (*Chuan Xiong*), 9g, Flos Carthami Tinctorii (*Hong Hua*), 9g, Radix Aconiti (*Chuan Wu*), 9g, Radix Aconiti Kusnezoffii (*Cao Wu*), 9g, Radix Clematidis Chinensis (*Wei Ling Xian*), 15g

D. Heat *bi*

Main symptoms: Joint aching and pain, redness, swelling, and a burning hot sensation at the site of pain. The pain is so acute that the spot cannot be touched. The sinews and vessels are stiff and tense and the joints are not able to move. When the area obtains chill, it relaxes. The tongue is red with a yellow coating, and the pulse is slippery and rapid.

Treatment principles: Clear heat and transform dampness, quicken the blood and open *bi*

Rx: Ramulus Cinnamomi (*Gui Zhi*), 4.5g, uncooked Gypsum Fibrosum (*Shi Gao*), 30g, Rhizoma Anemarrhenae (*Zhi Mu*), 9g, Cortex Phellodendri (*Huang Bai*), 9g, Semen Coicis Lachryma-jobi (*Mi Ren*), 30g, Radix Cyathulae (*Chuan Niu Xi*), 9g, Radix Stephaniae Tetrandrae (*Fang Ji*), 9g, Feces Bombycis Batryticati (*Jiang Sha*), 9g, Radix Rubrus Paeoniae Lactiflorae (*Chi Shao*), 9g, Cortex Radicis Moutan (*Dan Pi*), 9g, Radix Salviae Miltiorrhizae (*Dan Shen*), 15g, Caulis Lonicerae (*Ren Dong Teng*), 15g

E. Recalcitrant *bi*

Main symptoms: The joints of the bones are stiff and deformed. Their bending and stretching is inhibited. The aching and pain is intense. It is stopped (*i.e.* fixed) and its location does not vary. It may be numb or stiff and tense. It has not been cured even after enduring treatment. The tongue is purple with static patches, and the pulse is fine and choppy.

Treatment principles: Quicken the blood and transform stasis, warm yang and open *bi*

Rx: Semen Pruni Persicae (*Tao Ren*), 9g, Flos Carthami Tinctorii (*Hong Hua*), 9g, Radix Angelicae Sinensis (*Dang Gui*), 9g, Feces Trogopterori Seu Pteromi (*Wu Ling Zhi*), 9g, wine(-processed) Lumbricus (*Di Long*), 4.5g, Radix Ligustici Wallichii (*Chuan Xiong*), 9g, Resina Myrrhae (*Mo Yao*), 4.5g, Rhizoma Cyperi Rotundi (*Xiang Fu*), 9g, Radix Et Rhizoma Notopterygii (*Qiang Huo*), 9g, Radix Gentianae Macrophyllae (*Qin Jiao*), 9g, Radix Cyathula (*Chuan Niu Xi*), 9g, Radix Aconiti (*Chuan Wu*), 4.5g, Radix Aconiti Kusnezoffni (*Cao Wu*), 4.5g

Secret essentials

1. *Bi* means lack of free flow. Therefore, quickening the blood and transforming stasis enables the opening of the channels and the quickening of the network vessels. Hence these methods are most

suitable for this pathocondition. Pharmacological studies confirm that medicinals which quicken the blood and transform stasis produce a definite therapeutic effect on diseases which involve the immune system. My formula *Long Ma Ding Tong Dan* (Earthworm & Semen Strychnotis Stabilize Pain Elixir) has a curative rate of 90% in treating recalcitrant *bi*. The ingredients of these pills are: Semen Strychnotis (*Ma Qian Zi*), 30g, Guangdong Lumbricus (*Guang Di Long*), 3g, Buthus Martensi (*Quan Xie*), 3g, Scolopendra Subspinipes (*Wu Gong*), 3g. First one prepares the Semen Strychnotis. Then all the ingredients are ground into powder and made into 40 honey boluses. Each day, take 1 bolus.

2. In treating this condition, I like to use insects and worm medicinals, since they have the function of searching and picking out. The medicinals I commonly use are Catharsium Molossus (*Qiang Lang*), Eupolyphaga Seu Opisthoplatia (*Di Bei Chong*), Lumbricus (*Di Long*), Buthus Martensi (*Quan Xie*), and Scolopendra Subspinipes (*Wu Gong*). Their effects of dispersing swelling and stopping pain are marked. Snake flesh (*She Rou*) also has a specific effect on this pathocondition.

3. For joint swelling and distention, one can use Sichuan Rhizoma Dioscoreae Hypoglaucae (*Chuan Bi Xie*), uncooked Semen Coicis Lachryma-jobi (*Mi Ren*), and Rhizoma Smilacis Glabrae (*Tu Fu Ling*). For deformity of the joints, Nidus Vespae (*Feng Fang*) should be administered. In case of ceaseless pain, one can use large doses of *Shao Yao Gan Cao Tang* (Peony & Licorice Decoction). The amount of Peony varies from 15-20g, while that of Licorice ranges from 6-12g.

15. Atony patterns (*Wei Zheng*)

Atony patterns refer to looseness and slackness of the limbs, body, sinews, and vessels. The hands and feet are atonic, flaccid, and without strength. They cannot move at will. The muscles and flesh of diseased limbs mostly appear emaciated. If only the lower limbs are atonic and weak, this is called atonic feet. Similar conditions diagnosed by Western medicine, such as polyneuritis, myasthenia gravis, periodic paralysis, and progressive muscular dystrophy, may also be treated as atony patterns.

Disease causes, disease mechanisms

The ancients associated atony with the movement of the year (as in *wu yun liu qi* [five movements, six qi] theory). If heavy rain is followed by terrible summerheat, damp heat will brew and steam. The roots of grass and trees will mostly become rotten and the branches will become atonic (*i.e.*, withered). In years that earth is greatly excessive, people may be affected with atony. This is categorized as the external cause. In addition, if "thinking and longing are boundless but one's wishes are not obtained or if one manifests their lasciviousness externally and indulges in bedroom affairs too greatly, then the ancestral sinews will become slack and let loose and hence there is the onset of sinew atony." This is the internal cause of the arising of this disease. *Bi* patterns may also be transmuted into atony patterns. This is, in fact, due to stasis and obstruction of vessels and network vessels. The channels are thus not supplied and nourished by qi and blood. After a long time, atony will result from lack of use.

Treatment based on pattern discrimination

A. Damp heat steeping licentiously

Main symptoms: Atonic, weak, forceless limbs and body, possible swelling, possible itching, possible numbness, possible fever, desire for coolness and aversion to heat, heavy body, a yellow face, chest and epigastric glomus and fullness, red, astringent urination, a slimy tongue coating, and a soggy pulse

Treatment principles: Clear and transform dampness and heat, quicken the blood and raise the atonic

Rx: Rhizoma Atractylodis (*Cang Zhu*), 9g, Cortex Phellodendri (*Huang Bai*), 9g, Radix Gentianae Macrophyllae (*Qin Jiao*), 9g, Radix Achyranthis Bidentatae (*Niu Xi*), 9g, Radix Stephaniae Tetrandrae (*Fang Ji*), 9g, Radix Clematidis Chinensis (*Wei Ling Xian*), 15g, Flos Carthami Tinctorii (*Hong Hua*), 9g, Semen Coicis Lachryma-jobi (*Yi Ren*), 30g, Fructus Chaenomelis Lagenariae (*Mu Gua*), 9g, Radix Angelicae Pubescentis (*Du Huo*), 9g, Ramulus Mori Albi (*Sang Zhi*), 15g, Cortex Radicis Acanthopanacis (*Wu Jia Pi*), 9g

B. Liver/kidney deficiency & vacuity

Main symptoms: An initially slow onset of disease first manifesting as lower limb atony and weakness, gradual extension to the upper limbs, gradual desertion of the large flesh of the upper and lower legs, possible simultaneous impotence, premature ejaculation, vertigo and dizziness, a scarlet tongue, and a fine, rapid pulse

Treatment principles: Supplement and boost the liver and kidneys, quicken the blood and fill the marrow

Rx: Cortex Phellodendri (*Huang Bai*), 9g, Rhizoma Anemarrhenae (*Zhi Mu*), 9g, prepared Radix Rehmanniae (*Shu Di*), 15g, Plastrum Testudinis (*Gui Ban*), 15g, Cortex Radicis Moutan (*Dan Pi*), 9g, Radix Rubrus Paeoniae Lactiflorae (*Chi Shao*), 9g, Radix Salviae Miltiorrhizae (*Dan Shen*), 15g, Radix Angelicae Sinensis (*Dang Gui*), 9g, Radix Achyranthis Bidentatae (*Niu Xi*), 9g, Herba Cynomorii (*Suo Yang*), 9g, Herba Lycopodii (*Shen Jin Cao*), 15g, Radix Dipsaci (*Xu Duan*), 9g, Radix Asteris Tatarici (*Zi Wan*), 9g, Rhizoma Cimicifugae (*Sheng Ma*), 9g

C. Stasis obstruction of the vessels & network vessels

Main symptoms: Atony and weakness of the four limbs, bluish purple skin, typically numbness and insensitivity, occasional painful convulsions, a purple tongue, and a choppy pulse

Treatment principles: Boost the qi and nourish the constructive, quicken the blood and move stasis

Rx: Radix Rehmanniae (*Shu Di*), 15g, Radix Ligustici Wallichii (*Chuan Xiong*), 9g, Radix Rubrus Paeoniae Lactiflorae (*Chi Shao*), 9g, Radix Angelicae Sinensis (*Dang Gui*), 9g, Radix Salviae Miltiorrhizae (*Dan Shen*), 15g, Radix Astragali Membranacei (*Huang Qi*), 30g, Squama Manitis Pentadactylis (*Shan Jia*), 6g, Radix Clematidis Chinensis (*Wei Ling Xian*), 15g, Retinervus Citri Reticulatae (*Ju Luo*), 4.5g, Semen Pruni Persicae (*Tao Ren*), 9g, Flos Carthami Tinctorii (*Hong Hua*), 9g

Secret essentials

1. The ready-made medicine *Hu Qian Wan* (Crouching Tiger Pills) is indicated in this disease but sometimes is not effective. I often use a decoction of Herba Lycopodii (*Shen Jin Cao*), 120g, and Fructus Zizyphi Jujubae (*Hong Zao*), 7 pieces, to wash down *Hu Qian Wan*, and effects immediately respond.

2. In treating atony, I like to add Radix Asteris Tatarici (*Zi Wan*) and Rhizoma Cimicifugae (*Sheng Ma*). When Aster enters the lungs, the skin and flesh, sinews and bones of the five viscera will be nourished by lung fluids. The *Nei Jing (Inner Classic)* says, "Lung heat burns the lobes, and atony of the feet is engendered." This saying is clinically significant. The *Ben Jing (Root Classic, i.e., the Ben Cao Jing [Materia Medica Classic])* says that Aster is able to eliminate atony of the feet. Perhaps this is based on this idea. Spleen and stomach qi engenders the muscles and flesh and Cimicifuga is effective for activating the yang

vessels. The saying that "In treating atony, the *yang ming* alone should be selected" has far-reaching significance. If these two flavors (*i.e.*, medicinals) are added to the formula, they will raise up the atonic, vitalize the dilapidated, and open and free the channels and vessels. Thus, with half the effort, one may get double the effect.

8
Secret Essentials in the Treatment of Commonly Seen Geriatric Diseases

1. Lobar Pneumonia (*Da Ye Xing Fei Yan*)

Lobar pneumonia is caused by pneumococcus infection. Its chief clinical manifestations are chill, high fever, cough, chest pain, and spitting out rusty colored phlegm. In our national medicine (*i.e.*, TCM), this disease is discussed under dyspnea and cough (*chuan ke*), lung distention (*fei zhang*), damage by cold (*shang han*), and warm disease (*wen bing*) diseases and patterns. This disease may occur in all four seasons of the year but occurs most often in spring and winter. Although this disease usually occurs in young, strong adults, the elderly's weak bodily resistance and respiratory system often become predisposing factors for this disease. Further, its prognosis in the elderly is mostly unfavorable. According to relevant reports at home and abroad, the pneumonia bacillus ranks first in the death of the elderly due to infection. Therefore, one must address this disease with sufficient importance.

Disease causes, disease mechanisms

This disease is caused by invasion of external evils. The main evils are those of wind and warmth which enter the mouth and nose, invade the region of the lungs, and develop into this disease. This is what is meant by the saying, "Warm evils contracted above first invade the lungs." However, external invasion by wind cold may also cause this disease. In that case, depression transforms into heat. This heat then congests in the lungs. After external evils invade, they pass from the exterior to the interior and from the superficial part to the deep region. This generally develops according to the warm disease theory of defensive, qi, constructive, and blood. At first, evils are in the lung defensive and an exterior pattern and lung symptoms appear. Then they enter the qi aspect and there is great heat. At this stage, symptoms of phlegm heat congesting in the lungs appear. If the disease develops further, evils enter and burn the constructive. If severe, the righteous may not vanquish these evils. Evil heat may thus damage true yin and true yang. In that case, yin fluids are consumed and exhausted or yang qi may become vacuous and desert.

Treatment based on pattern discrimination

A. Evils assailing lung defensive

Main symptoms: Aversion to cold, fever, cough, chest pain, discomfort in the brain, dry mouth leading to drinking, sides of the tongue inflamed and red, a thin, white or thin, yellow tongue coating, and a floating, rapid pulse

Treatment principles: Use acrid and cool medicinals to resolve the exterior, clear and transform phlegm stasis

Rx: Radix Et Rhizoma Polygoni Cymosi (*Kai Jin Suo*), 30g, Herba Houttuyniae Cordatae (*Yu Xing Cao*), 30g, Rhizoma Polygoni Cuspidati (*Hu Zhang*), 15g, Semen Pruni Persicae (*Tao Ren*), 9g, Semen Benincasae Hispidae (*Dong Gua Zi*), 10g, Retinervus Fasciculoris Citri Reticulatae (*Ju Luo*), 3g, Flos Lonicerae Japonicae (*Yin Hua*), 9g, Fructus Forsythiae Suspensae (*Lian Qiao*), 9g, Semen Pruni Armeniacae (*Xing Ren*), 9g, Semen Coicis Lachryma-jobi (*Ku Mi Ren*), 9g, Radix Salviae Miltiorrhizae (*Dan Shen*), 9g

B. Phlegm heat congesting the lungs

Main symptoms: Fever but no cold or possible cold shivering, oral thirst, cough, chest pain, yellow, pasty phlegm which may contain threads of blood or possibly an iron-rust color, flaring nostrils, hard breathing, yellow urine, a dry tongue with a yellow coating, and a surging, large or slippery rapid pulse

Treatment principles: Clear heat and dispel stasis, diffuse the lungs and transform phlegm

Rx: Herba Ephedrae (*Ma Huang*), 6g, Semen Pruni Armeniacae (*Xing Ren*), 9g, Gypsum Fibrosum (*Shi Gao*), 30g, uncooked Radix Glycyrrhizae (*Gan Cao*), 3g, Semen Lepidii (*Ting Li Zi*), 9g, Semen Pruni Persicae (*Tao Ren*), 9g, Herba Houttuyniae Cordatae (*Yu Xing Cao*), 30g, Radix Scutellariae Baicalensis (*Huang Qin*), 9g, Radix Rubrus Paeoniae Lactiflorae (*Chi Shao*), 9g, *Dai Ge San* (Indigo & Clam Shell)[3], 9g, wrapped during decoction

C. Qi & yin dual vacuity, phlegm & heat joining and contending

Main symptoms: Cough, low fever, spiritual fatigue, poor appetite, spontaneous perspiration, heart vexation, a red tongue with a thin coating, and a fine, rapid pulse

Treatment principles: Boost the qi and nourish yin, transform phlegm and dispel stasis

Rx: Radix Adenophorae Strictae (*Nan Sha Shen*), 9g, Radix Glehniae Littoralis (*Bei Sha Shen*), 9g, Tuber Ophiopogonis Japonicae (*Mai Dong*), 9g, Semen Benincasae Hispidae (*Dong Gua Zi*), 9g, Semen Coicis Lachryma-jobi (*Yi Ren*), 15g, Semen Pruni Persicae (*Tao Ren*), 9g, Concha Arcae (*Wa Leng Zi*), 15g, Folium Lophatheri Gracilis (*Dan Zhu Ye*), 9g, Cortex Radicis Moutan (*Dan Pi*), 9g, Cortex Radicis Lycii (*Di Gu Pi*), 9g, fresh Rhizoma Phragmitis Communis (*Lu Gen*), 30g

D. Original qi vacuity desertion, yin & yang dissociated

Main symptoms: A somber white complexion, great perspiration dribbling and dripping, inversion chill of the four limbs, a fine, minute

---

[3] This is a patent medicine composed of: Calcined Concha Cyclinae (*Ge Ke*), 180 g., and Pulvis Indigonis (*Qing Dai*), 18 g.

or bound, regularly interrupted pulse. This is a critical sign of evil toxins internally falling.

Treatment principles: Secure yang and stem counterflow, quicken the blood and transform stasis

Rx: Radix Codonopsis Pilosulae (*Dang Shen*), 30g, Radix Lateralis Praeparatus Aconiti Carmichaeli (*Fu Pian*), 9g, Ramulus Cinnamomi (*Gui Zhi*), 4.5g, calcined Os Draconis (*Long Gu*), 30g, calcined Concha Ostreae (*Mu Li*), 30g, Tuber Ophiopogonis Japonicae (*Mai Dong*), 9g, Fructus Schizandrae Chinensis (*Wu Wei Zi*), 9g, Flos Carthami Tinctorii (*Hong Hua*), 9g, Radix Salviae Miltiorrhizae (*Dan Shen*), 15g, Radix Rubrus Paeoniae Lactiflorae (*Chi Shao*), 9g, mix-fried Radix Glycyrrhizae (*Zhi Gan Cao*), 4.5g

Secret Essentials

1. Pneumonia which lasts a long time without resolution is mostly due to lung qi insufficiency. Therefore, use Radix Astragali Membranacei (*Huang Qi*), 30g, and Folium Mahoniae (*Gong Lao Ye*), 9g, decocted in water and administered 1 *ji* per day.

2. If high fever in pneumonia does not recede, it is all right to use *Zi Xue Dan* (Purple Snow Elixir), 1g 2-3 times per day.

3. In the elderly, it is necessary to treat both branch and root at the same time. If the righteous does not vanquish evils, then infectious shock may occur. Therefore, taking the root into account, one should add to the chosen formula Radix Adenophorae Strictae (*Nan Sha Shen*), Radix Glehniae Littoralis (*Bei Sha Shen*), Folium Mahoniae (*Gong Lao Ye*), Tuber Ophiopogonis Japonicae (*Mai Dong*), and Radix Pseudostellariae (*Tai Zi Shen*).

4. For those with yin vacuity, correspondingly one should enrich and nourish yin. In such cases, the righteous qi is insufficient, electrolytes are confused, and treatment with medicinals is not able to fully display

its effects. Thus it is sometimes necessary to add Radix Panacis Quinquefolii (*Yang Shen*), Herba Dendrobii (*Shi Hu*), Radix Trichosanthis Kirlowii (*Hua Fen*), Tuber Ophiopogonis Japonicae (*Mai Dong*), and Rhizoma Phragmitis Communis (*Lu Gen*) in order that the yin aspect may be restored. This is a key point for determining the subsequent course of this disease.

2. Hypertension (*Gao Xue Ya*)

Hypertension is one of the commonly seen diseases in the elderly. In the hypertensive patient, there is great danger of developing cardiac and/or cerebral vascular complications. Careful treatment will not only reduce the incidence of serious cardiac and cerebral complications and lower the death and disability rate but can also lengthen longevity and improve the life of the aged.

Senile hypertension means that, in those over 65, the diastolic pressure is over 13 Kpa, the systolic pressure is over 21 Kpa, or the values of both of these exceed the above limits. In TCM, this disease is categorized as vertigo and dizziness (*xuan yun*), liver yang (*gan yang*), and liver wind (*gan feng*).

Disease causes, disease mechanisms

The chief cause of this disease is loss of regulation of the emotions and orientation and lack of discipline in drinking and eating. There may be long-standing nervous tension, irritation, anger, worry, and over-thinking. Thus there is liver qi depression and stagnation with enduring depression transforming into fire. It is also possible that taxation and damage beyond limit may lead to kidney yin vacuity and deficiency. The liver thus loses its nourishment and yin does not restrain yang. Hence liver yang becomes hyperactive above. If one eats without restraint sweet, fatty foods or drinks alcohol beyond limit, dampness and turbidity will gather and check. Enduring brewing transforms into fire, fluids are stewed into phlegm, and phlegm turbidity comes with liver fire to harass above.

Under the influence of the above-mentioned various factors, the dispersion and growth of yin and yang in the human body lose their regulation. In particular, the liver and kidney yin and yang lose their regulation, giving rise to the pathological phenomena of vacuity below and repletion above. Thus one may see headache, dizziness, and tinnitus. Kidney disease may reach the heart, causing loss of communication between the heart and kidneys. Hence one may also see heart palpitations, poor memory, and insomnia. If liver wind enters the network vessels, one may see numbness in the four limbs and, if serious, deviation of eyes and mouth. If liver fire counterflows upward, the eyes may be red and the patient likes to get angry. If wind and fire fan each other, blood will follow qi and be upborne. This disturbs the spirit brilliance and mists the clear portals. It may further bring about the serious consequences of wind stroke and syncope.

Treatment based on pattern discrimination

A. Liver fire hyperactivity & exuberance

Main symptoms: Headache, vertigo and dizziness, a red face, red eyes, a bitter taste in the mouth, vexation and agitation, constipation, yellow urination, a red tongue with a yellow coating, and a wiry, large pulse

Treatment principles: Level the liver and drain fire, quicken the blood and transform stasis

Rx: Radix Gentianae Scabrae (*Long Dan Cao*), 9g, Rhizoma Coptidis Chinensis (*Huang Lian*), 2.4g, Radix Scutellariae Baicalensis (*Huang Qin*), 9g, Concha Haliotidis (*Shi Jue Ming*), 30g, Flos Chrysanthemi Morifolii (*Ju Hua*), 9g, Radix Salviae Miltiorrhizae (*Dan Shen*), 15g, Cortex Radicis Moutan (*Dan Pi*), 9g, Semen Pruni Persicae (*Tao Ren*), 9g, Herba Leonuri Heterophylli (*Yi Mu Cao*), 30g, Radix Achyranthis Bidentatae (*Niu Xi*), 9g, Semen Cassiae Torae (*Jue Ming Zi*), 30g, Radix Ligustici Wallichii (*Chuan Xiong*), 6g

B. Yin vacuity, yang hyperactivity

Main symptoms: Dizziness, headache, low back and knee soreness and weakness, tinnitus, poor memory, vexatious heat in the five hearts, heart palpitations, loss of sleep, a red tongue with a thin coating, and a wiry, rapid pulse

Treatment principles: Foster yin and subdue yang, quicken the blood and transform stasis

Rx: Fructus Lycii Chinensis (*Qi Zi*), 9g, Flos Chrysanthemi Morifolii (*Ju Hua*), 9g, Fructus Corni Officinalis (*Yu Rou*), 6g, Rhizoma Alismatis (*Ze Xie*), 9g, uncooked Radix Rehmanniae (*Sheng Di*), 15g, Cortex Radicis Moutan (*Dan Pi*), 9g, Radix Dioscoreae Oppositae (*Shan Yao*), 9g, Sclerotium Poriae Cocos (*Fu Ling*), 9g, Carapax Amydae Sinensis (*Bie Jia*), 15g, Radix Rubrus Paeoniae Lactiflorae (*Chi Shao*), 9g, Radix Ligustici Wallichii (*Chuan Xiong*), 6g, Concha Margaritiferae (*Zhen Zhu Mu*), 30g

C. Yin & yang dual vacuity

Major symptoms: Dizziness, headache, tinnitus, heart palpitations, movement stirs rapid breathing, low back, knee, and feet weakness, loss of sleep, excessive dreams, a red tongue or a pale red tongue with white coating, and a wiry, fine pulse

Treatment principles: Foster yin and aid yang, quicken the blood and transform stasis

Rx: Rhizoma Anemarrhenae (*Zhi Mu*), 9g, Cortex Phellodendri (*Huang Bai*), 9g, Rhizoma Curculiginis Orchoidis (*Xian Mao*), 9g, Herba Epimedii (*Xian Ling Pi*), 9g, Radix Angelicae Sinensis (*Dang Gui*), 9g, Radix Morindae Officinalis (*Ba Ji Tian*), 9g, Spica Prunellae Vulgaris (*Xia Ku Cao*), 9g, Radix Rubrus Paeoniae Lactiflorae (*Chi Shao*), 15g, Herba Leonuri Heterophylli (*Yi Mu Cao*), 30g

D. Phlegm dampness congestion & exuberance

Major symptoms: Dizziness, headache, heavy head, chest oppression, heart palpitations, scanty appetite, nausea and vomiting of phlegmy fluids, a dark tongue with a slimy coating, and a mostly soggy, slippery pulse

Treatment principles: Eliminate phlegm and transform dampness, move the blood and clear the channels

Rx: Rhizoma Pinelliae Ternatae (*Ban Xia*), 9g, Rhizoma Gastrodiae Elatae (*Tian Ma*), 4.5g, Rhizoma Atractylodis Macrocephalae (*Bai Zhu*), 9g, Ramulus Uncariae Cum Uncis (*Gou Teng*), 15g, Fructus Crataegi (*Shan Zha*), 9g, uncooked Pollen Typhae (*Pu Huang*), 9g, wrapped during decoction, Radix Ligustici Wallichii (*Chuan Xiong*), 9g, Semen Cassiae Torae (*Jue Ming Zi*), 30g, Sclerotium Poriae Cocos (*Fu Ling*), 9g, bile(-processed) Rhizoma Arisaematis (*Dan Xing*), 9g, Fructus Immaturus Citri Seu Ponciri (*Zhi Shi*), 9g, Radix Salviae Miltiorrhizae (*Dan Shen*), 15g

Secret Essentials

1. Observation reveals that the tongue of those who are hypertensive is mostly dark red. This pathological change is due to the constriction of the arteries and increase in the peripheral vascular resistance. This has a close relationship with static blood. I regularly administer Herba Sargassii (*Hai Zao*), Rhizoma Curcumae Zedoariae (*E Zhu*), 9g @, in decoction. This is able to downbear the pressure, increase blood flow, and soften the blood vessels.

2. Decoct Semen Plantaginis (*Che Qian Zi*), 30g, and 2 drinks per day. This has a marked effect in reducing diastolic pressure.

3. Heart Disease due to Coronary Artery Atherosclerosis (*Guan Zhuang Dong Mai Zhou Yang Ying Hua Xing Xin Zang Bing*)

Heart disease due to coronary artery atherosclerosis is called, for short, coronary heart disease. Because its main symptom is acute chest pain, it corresponds to chest *bi* (*xiong bi*), true heart pain (*zhen xin tong*), and inversion heart pain (*jue xin tong*) in TCM. If heart pain is severe, the greenish blue (*i.e.*, cyanotic) color of the hands and feet may extend to the joints. As it is recorded:

> If onset is in the morning, death at night. If onset is at night, death in the morning.

This is one of the three main diseases that account for the death of the elderly.

Disease causes, disease mechanisms

Heart yang may be devitalized. In addition, cold evils may be contracted. Thus yin cold is exuberant in the temple of the chest. Yang qi loses its diffusion, and cold congeals in the blood vessels. It is also possible that strong wine and thick flavors cause detriment to and damage the spleen and stomach. Phlegm turbidity and fatty substances are engendered internally. Thus the transportation and movement of qi and blood is obstructed and hindered. Or, due to emotional depression, qi may stagnate in the upper burner. Hence chest yang loses its outspreading and the blood vessels are not harmonious. Further, the qi and yin of the elderly are both debilitated. The blood vessels are blocked and obstructed and the heart loses its nourishment. As Zhang Zhongjing pointed out, "Yang is minute, and yin is wiry." This is the most important disease mechanism in the occurrence of heart pain.

Treatment based on pattern discrimination

A. Chest yang *bi* & obstruction

Main symptoms: Heart pain, often induced by cold, shortness of breath, blockage and oppression within the chest, in severe cases, heart pain radiating to the upper back and upper back pain extending to the chest, a slimy tongue coating, and a wiry, slippery pulse

Treatment principles: Open yang and diffuse *bi*, quicken the blood and transform stasis

Rx: Fructus Trichosanthis Kirlowii (*Gua Lou*), 9g, Bulbus Allii Macrostemi (*Xie Bai*), 9g, Ramulus Cinnamomi (*Gui Zhi*), 4.5g, Radix Ligustici Wallichii (*Chuan Xiong*), 9g, uncooked Pollen Typhae (*Pu Huang*), 9g, wrapped during decoction, uncooked Rhizoma Cyperi Rotundi (*Xiang Fu*), 9g, Rhizoma Pinelliae Ternatae (*Ban Xia*), 9g, Radix Salviae Miltiorrhizae (*Dan Shen*), 15g, Flos Carthami Tinctorii (*Hong Hua*), 9g, powdered Sanguis Draconis (*Xue Jie*), 1.5g, powdered Radix Pseudoginseng (*San Qi*), 1.5g. (These two powders are mixed together and chased down by the other decocted medicinals have been decocted.)

B. Heart vessel stasis & obstruction

Main symptoms: Heart and chest piercing pain, both lateral costal regions distended and full, shortness of breath, heart vexation, restlessness, a dark red tongue or purple and dark with static patches, bluish purple veins at the root of the tongue, and a wiry, choppy pulse

Treatment principles: Quicken the blood and transform stasis, open the vessels and stop pain

Rx: Radix Salviae Miltiorrhizae (*Dan Shen*), 15g, Semen Pruni Persicae (*Tao Ren*), 9g, Radix Bupleuri (*Chai Hu*), 9g, Radix Ligustici Wallichii (*Chuan Xiong*), 9g, *Shi Xiao San* (Sudden Smile Powder), 9g, Radix Angelicae Sinensis (*Dang Gui*), 9g, Radix Rubrus Paeoniae Lactiflorae

(*Chi Shao*), 9g, Radix Albus Paeoniae Lactiflorae (*Bai Shao*), 9g, clear mix-fried Radix Glycyrrhizae (*Qing Zhi Cao*), 4.5g, Flos Carthami Tinctorii (*Hong Hua*), 9g, Ramulus Cinnamomi (*Gui Zhi*), 4.5g.

C. Phlegm turbidity internally obstructing

Main symptoms: Chest oppression or chest pain, a fat body, bodily heaviness, lack of strength, extremely excessive phlegm, pasty slime within the mouth, a thick, slimy or filthy, turbid tongue coating, and a slippery, replete pulse

Treatment principles: Use fragrant and aromatic medicinals to transform turbidity, disinhibit phlegm and dispel stasis

Rx: Ginger(-processed) Rhizoma Coptidis Chinensis (*Huang Lian*), 2.4g, Cortex Magnoliae Officinalis (*Chuan Po*), 6g, Tuber Curcumae (*Yu Jin*), 9g, Rhizoma Acori Graminei (*Chang Pu*), 9g, Radix Polygalae Tenuifoliae (*Yuan Zhi*), 9g, Rhizoma Pinelliae Ternatae (*Ban Xia*), 9g, Fructus Immaturus Citri Seu Ponciri (*Zhi Shi*), 9g, Lignum Santali Albi (*Tan Xiang*), 1.5g, Fructus Piperis Longi (*Pi Ba*), Radix Ligustici Wallichii (*Chuan Xiong*), 9g, Fructus Crataegi (*Zha Rou*), 9g, Flos Carthami Tinctorii (*Hong Hua*), 9g

D. Qi & yin dual deficiency

Main symptoms: Heart pain, shortness of breath, heart palpitations, spontaneous perspiration, a dry mouth with scant fluids, dizziness, insomnia, a red tongue with no coating, in severe cases a peeled coating, and a fine, rapid or bound, regularly interrupted pulse

Treatment principles: Radix Pseudostellariae (*Tai Zi Shen*), 15g, Radix Astragali Membranacei (*Huang Qi*), 15g, Radix Puerariae (*Ge Gen*), 9g, Radix Salviae Miltiorrhizae (*Dan Shen*), 15g, Semen Cassiae Torae (*Jue Ming Zi*), 30g, Fructus Crataegi (*Shan Zha*), 9g, Radix Rubrus Paeoniae Lactiflorae (*Chi Shao*), 9g, Fructus Schizandrae Chinensis (*Wu Wei Zi*), 6g, Tuber Ophiopogonis Japonicae (*Mai Dong*),

9g, Concha Margaritifera (*Zhen Zhu Mu*), 30g, Rhizoma Gastrodiae Elatae (*Tian Ma*), 4.5g

E. Kidney yang vacuity weakness

Main symptoms: Heart palpitations and throbbing, heart pain, shortness of breath, spiritual fatigue, fear of cold, exacerbation of heart pain when exposed to chill, lack of warmth in the four limbs, low back soreness and foot weakness, a pale but dark tongue with a white coating, and a deep and fine or bound, regularly irregular pulse

Treatment principles: Radix Lateralis Praeparatus Aconiti Carmichaeli (*Fu Pian*), 6g, Ramulus Cinnamomi (*Gui Zhi*), 4.5g, uncooked Radix Rehmanniae (*Sheng Di*), 15g, Fructus Corni Officinalis (*Yu Rou*), 9g, Radix Dioscoreae Oppositae (*Shan Yao*), 9g, Sclerotium Poriae Cocos (*Fu Ling*), 9g, Rhizoma Alismatis (*Ze Xie*), 9g, Cortex Radicis Moutan (*Dan Pi*), 9g, Radix Ligustici Wallichii (*Chuan Xiong*), 9g, Radix Angelicae Sinensis (*Dang Gui*), 9g, Radix Rubrus Paeoniae Lactiflorae (*Chi Shao*), 15g

F. Yang vacuity tending to desertion

Main symptoms: Heart pain, shortness of breath, great perspiration dribbling and dripping, inversion chill of the four limbs, bluish purple nails, a somber white complexion, danger of inversion desertion, a dark tongue with a white coating, and a deep, fine, tending to expire pulse

Treatment principles: Return yang and secure desertion, quicken the blood and stem counterflow

Rx: Radix Panacis Ginseng (*Ren Shen*), 9g, Radix Lateralis Praeparatus Aconiti Carmichaeli (*Fu Zi*), 9g, Os Draconis (*Long Gu*), 30g, Concha Ostreae (*Mu Li*),30g, Ramulus Cinnamomi (*Gui Zhi*), 4.5g, Radix Albus Paeoniae Lactiflorae (*Bai Shao*), 9g, mix-fried Radix Glycyrrhizae (*Zhi Gan Cao*), 4.5g, Radix Ligustici Wallichii (*Chuan Xiong*), 9g, Flos

Carthami Tinctorii (*Hong Hua*), 9g, Radix Rubrus Paeoniae Lactiflorae (*Chi Shao*), 9g, Semen Pruni Persicae (*Tao Ren*), 9g

Secret Essentials

1. The disease mechanism of coronary heart disease lies in "yang deficiency, yin congelation." If one simply resolves congelation, one can achieve effects only for a time. Therefore, it is necessary to warm and open yang at the same time. Aconite is the medicinal of first choice.

2. Powdered Sanguis Draconis (*Xue Jie*) and powdered Radix Pseudo-ginseng (*San Qi*), 1.5g @, are mixed evenly and administered. In treating angina pectoris, these medicinals produce prompt effects.

3. *Heng Fa Sheng Fang* (Balancing Method Sagelike Formula) can prevent and treat this disease. It is better than typically breaking the qi and quickening the blood. It has the function of securing the root and clearing the source. In particular, it is beneficial for restoring over-taxed heart muscles which have sustained detriment. Method of administration: 1 packet each time, 1 time per day.

4. Acupuncture is effective in treating heart pain. Body acupuncture: *Tan Zhong* (CV 17), *Nei Guan* (Per 6), and *Zu San Li* (St 36). Retain the needles for 20 minutes. Twist and rotate them every 5 minutes. Ear acupuncture: *Xin* (Heart), *Shen Men* (Spirit Gate), and *Pi Zhi Xia* (Subcortex).

4. Cerebral Stroke (*Nao Zu Zhong*)

Cerebral stroke is popularly known as wind stroke. It is categorized as nerve damage in a specific region of the brain due to acute, non-traumatic obstruction to the blood flow. Its clinical manifestations are sudden attack, obstruction of consciousness, and hemiplegia. This disease is categorized as wind stroke (*zhong feng*), death stroke (*zu zhong*), and dumbness disease (*ye fei*) in our national medicine (*i.e.*, TCM).

Disease causes, disease mechanisms

Hemorrhagic cerebral vascular disease is mainly due to cerebral hemorrhage in turn due to hypertension. Cerebral vascular disease due to local anemia is mainly due to cerebral thrombosis, cerebral embolism, and occurrence of temporary lack of blood to the brain. This disease is usually caused by worry, over-thinking, irritation, anger, or lack of restraint in alcohol, eating rich, fatty foods, damage due to bedroom affairs, or taxation beyond limit resulting in yin deficiency below. Once the five orientations are carried to an extreme, liver yang cannot be controlled and internal wind is sent whirling and is stirred. Qi and blood counterflow, chaotically mixed with phlegm and fire. They traverse the channels and vessels, misting the portals of the heart and causing sudden falling in a faint and hemiplegia. During the acute stage of this disease, the condition is very serious, manifesting the symptoms of "internal blockage, external desertion." It often threatens one's life destiny. During the recovery stage, qi vacuity and blood stasis are the principal contradictions.

Treatment based on pattern discrimination

A. Blockage pattern

Main symptoms: The patient suddenly falls down in a faint, unconscious of human affairs. The teeth are tightly closed. The mouth is silent and not open. The two hands are tightly clenched. There is constipation and urinary retention. The limbs are stiff. Clinically, stoke may be divided into yang blockage and yin blockage. In yang blockage, the face is red and the body is hot. There is forceful breathing, bad breath, vexation, worry, and restlessness. The tongue coating is yellow and slimy, and the pulse is wiry, slippery, and rapid. In yin blockage, the face is white while the lips are dark. The patient lies still and is not vexed. The four limbs are not warm. Phlegm drool congests and is exuberant. The tongue coating is white and slimy, and the pulse is deep, slippery, and relaxed (retarded).

Treatment principles for yang blockage: Clear the liver and search wind, open the portals and transform stasis

Rx: Powdered Cornu Antelopis Saigae Tataricae (*Ling Yang Jiao*), 1.5g, Rhizoma Acori Graminei (*Chang Pu*), 12g, uncooked Radix Et Rhizoma Rhei (*Jun*), 9g, Dens Draconis (*Long Chi*), 30g, Concretio Silicea Bambusae (*Tian Zhu Huang*), 9g, Herba Menthae Haplocalycis (*Bo He*), 4.5g, Radix Scutellariae Baicalensis (*Huang Qin*), 9g, Ramulus Uncariae Cum Uncis (*Gou Teng*), 15g, Rhizoma Coptidis Chinensis (*Chuan Lian*), 3g, Calcitum (*Han Shui Shi*), 30g, *An Gong Niu Huang Wan* (Quiet the Palace Bezoar Pills), 1 bolus, dissolved and taken

Treatment principles for yin blockage: Break up phlegm and search wind, open the portals and transform stasis

Rx: *Su He Xiang Wan* (Styrax Pills), 1 bolus, taken orally dissolved in warm water. Wait a bit and then use the following formula: Flos Carthami Tinctorii (*Hong Hua*), 9g, Semen Pruni Persicae (*Tao Ren*), 9g, Retinervus Fascicularis Citri Reticulatae (*Ju Luo*), 4.5g, Rhizoma Acori Graminei (*Chang Pu*), 9g, Radix Ligustici Wallichii (*Chuan Xiong*), 9g, Radix Rubrus Paeoniae Lactiflorae (*Chi Shao*), 9g, ginger(-processed) Rhizoma Pinelliae Ternatae (*Ban Xia*), 9g, Ramulus Cinnamomi (*Gui Zhi*), 6g, Tuber Curcumae (*Yu Jin*), 9g, Fructus Immaturus Citri Seu Ponciri (*Zhi Shi*), 9g, Rhizoma Arisaematis (*Nan Xing*), 9g

Acupuncture: Needle *Ren Zhong* (GV 26), *Shi Xuan* (Extra points), *Tai Chong* (Liv 3), and *Feng Long* (St 40) with strong needle stimulation.

B. Desertion pattern

Main symptoms: If blockage pattern is not rescued with force or if the condition of the disease deteriorates, then it will develop into desertion pattern. The manifestations are blockage of the eyes, opening of the mouth, snoring, faint breathing, hands spread open, chilled limbs, sweat like oil, spontaneous urination. an atonic tongue, and a minute pulse tending to expiry

Treatment principles: Boost the qi and quicken the blood, return yang and stem yin

Rx: Radix Lateralis Praeparatus Aconiti Carmichaeli (*Fu Pian*), 9g, dry Rhizoma Zingiberis (*Gan Jiang*), 2.4g, Rhizoma Atractylodis Macrocephalae (*Bai Zhu*), 9g, Radix Glycyrrhizae (*Gan Cao*), 3g, Semen Pruni Persicae (*Tao Ren*), 9g, Flos Carthami Tinctorii (*Hong Hua*), 9g, Radix Panacis Ginseng (*Ren Shen*), 9g, Tuber Ophiopogonis Japonicae (*Mai Dong*), 9g, Fructus Schizandrae Chinensis (*Wu Wei Zi*), 9g

C. Hemiplegia

Main symptoms: The movement of the limbs on one side of the body are not able to be consciously controlled. In mild cases, there is numbness. In severe cases, there is complete loss of consciousness. The body and limbs are paralyzed and weak. The tongue is purple and dark and the tongue coating is white and slimy. The pulse is slippery, relaxed (retarded), and forceless.

Treatment principles: Boost the qi and transform stasis, dispel wind and eliminate phlegm

Rx: Radix Astragali Membranacei (*Huang Qi*), 60g, Radix Ligustici Wallichii (*Chuan Xiong*), 9g, Radix Rubrus Paeoniae Lactiflorae (*Chi Shao*), 9g, Flos Carthami Tinctorii (*Hong Hua*), 9g, wine(-processed) Lumbricus (*Di Long*), 6g, Radix Angelicae Sinensis (*Dang Gui*), 9g, Herba Siegesbeckiae (*Xi Xian Cao*), 15g, Hirudo (*Shui Zhi*), 3g, uncooked Pollen Typhae (*Pu Huang*), 9g, Rhizoma Acori Graminei (*Chang Pu*), 9g, Radix Gentianae Macrophyllae (*Qin Jiao*), 9g

D. Speech obstructed & astringed

Main symptoms: The tongue does not move freely. Speech is not clear. Drool flows by itself. The tongue is mostly wry and deviated. The tongue coating is thin and slimy. The pulse is slippery and relaxed (retarded).

Treatment principles: Break up phlegm and disinhibit the portals, quicken the blood and transform stasis

Rhizoma Gastrodiae Elatae (*Tian Ma*), 4.5g, powdered Buthus Martensi (*Quan Xie*), 1.5g, Rhizoma Typhonii (*Bai Fu Zi*), 9g, bile(-processed) Rhizoma Arisaematis (*Dan Xing*), 9g, Fructus Immaturus Citri Seu Ponciri (*Zhi Shi*), 9g, Fructus Trichosanthis Kirlowii (*Quan Gua Lou*), 12g, Concretio Silicea Bambusae (*Tian Zhu Huang*), 9g, Rhizoma Acori Graminei (*Chang Pu*), 9g, Radix Polygalae Tenuifoliae (*Yuan Zhi*), 9g, Radix Salviae Miltiorrhizae (*Dan Shen*), 15g, Radix Ligustici Wallichii (*Chuan Xiong*), 9g, Flos Carthami Tinctorii (*Hong Hua*), 9g, Hirudo (*Shui Zhi*), 3g

Secret Essentials

1. The discovery that blood stasis is the chief mechanism in the cause of cerebral stroke has made a great development in the theoretical basis of TCM. Whether it is wind stroke due to lack of blood or hemorrhagic wind stroke, there is usually stasis in the cerebral region. Therefore, clinically, when using medicinals, one should not forget to transform stasis since it is the crux which influences the turning point in this disease. Hemorrhagic wind stroke is by no means an exception. Some people think that, during the stage of acute attack, it is not proper to quicken the blood and transform stasis. In fact, where there is hemorrhage, there must be stasis. Only when static is cleared and eliminated can the function of the clear spirit be restored. In TCM, there are numerous treatment methods and formulas for the treatment of this disease. Therefore, we should not feel humble.

2. In treating acute wind stroke, one must be innovative when it comes to the form of dosage of medicinals. We must race against time in order to find new ways to use old medicinals. The Beijing College of TCM has added medicinals for quickening the blood and transforming stasis to the ancient formula *An Gong Niu Huang Wan* (Quiet the Palace Bezoar Pills). This has been manufactured for intravenous infusion as *Qing Kai Ling Fa She Ye* (Clearing & Opening Magical Method Injectable Fluid). Its clinical effects are quite satisfactory. This is really a good innovation.

3. I have recently used uncooked Pollen Typhae (*Pu Huang*), Radix Astragali Membranacei (*Huang Qi*), and Radix Ligustici Wallichii (*Chuan Xiong*) to prepare *Zhong Feng Yu Fang Chong Ji* (Wind Stroke Prevention Soluble Granules). One packet is taken each time, 2 times per day. It is taken dissolved in hot water. This medicine is designed to treat qi and blood stasis and obstruction. This is worthy of further exploration.

4. *Heng Fa Sheng Fang* (Balancing Method Sagelike Formula) is indicated for the sequelae of wind stroke, such as hemiplegia, hemianaesthia, aphasia, deviation of eyes and mouth, spirit orientation loss of normalcy, spirit manner rigid and wooden, and convulsive tremors of the limbs and body. One packet is taken each time, 1 time per day.

5. Diabetes Mellitus (*Tang Niao Bing*)

In the medical history of the world, the earliest knowledge of this disease is found in TCM. In the *Nei Jing (Inner Classic)*, there are already records on *xiao ke* or wasting and thirst, including discussions of the symptoms and causes of this disease. The *Jin Gui Yao Lue (Essential Prescriptions from the Golden Chamber)* advanced all the more clearly the theory that this disease is characterized by "three polys". These are "dispersion of grain" (*i.e.*, polyphagia), "drinking a peck" (*i.e.*, polydipsia), and "urinating a peck" (*i.e.*, polyuria). Many physicians in different dynasties further clarified this disease. For instance, the *Zhu Bing Yuan Hou Lun (Treatise on the Origins & Symptoms of Various Diseases)* says, "This disease often originates from *yong* and *ju*". Liu Wan-su said, "Those with wasting and thirsting often also go deaf or blind." Thus he had already discussed the complications of diabetes mellitus. The *Gu Jin Yi Tong (Ancient & Modern Medicine Gathered Together)* further mentions that the treatment of this disease responds to "bland, enriching flavors." All these statements reflect the advanced character of our national medical theory (*i.e.*, TCM).

The clinical course or progression of senile diabetes mellitus is rather slow. Patients with marked symptoms of the "three polys" only account for one fourth of elderly diabetics, while complications are predominant. Therefore, this disease is often overlooked in diagnosis. On the other hand, elderly diabetics usually have painless cardiac infarction and diabetic renal diseases. Hence hypertonic coma can occur suddenly attended by its consequent dangers.

Disease causes, disease mechanisms

Yin fluid deficiency and detriment and dry heat internally engendered are the chief disease mechanisms of diabetes mellitus. The causative factors may be roughly as follows: Prolonged and excessive eating of fats and sweets, drinking strong wine (*i.e.*, alcohol), and eating thick flavors may cause accumulation in the stomach which produces internal heat. This disperses grains and consumes fluids. It is also possible for long-term emotional depression to result in fire heat accumulating internally. This consumes and damages yin fluids. In addition, lack of discipline in bedroom affairs can cause kidney essence deficiency and detriment. Vacuity fire is made even stronger. This disease may also be caused by recklessly using strengthening yang and warm, dry substances. Dry heat is the branch, while yin vacuity is the root. Branch and root serve as cause and effect for each other.

Treatment based on pattern discrimination

A. Upper wasting: Lung heat, fluids damaged

Main symptoms: Vexatious thirst, polydipsia, a dry mouth and tongue, frequent urination, amount excessive, red tongue edges and tip, a thin, yellow tongue coating, and a surging, rapid pulse

Treatment principles: Clear heat and moisten the lungs, engender fluids and quicken the blood

Rx: Radix Scrophulariae Ningpoensis (*Xuan Shen*), 15g, Tuber Ophiopogonis Japonicae (*Mai Dong*), 9g, Tuber Asparagi Cochinensis (*Tian Dong*), 9g, uncooked Radix Rehmanniae (*Sheng Di*), 15g, Herba Dendrobii (*Shi Hu*), 9g, Rhizoma Anemarrhenae (*Zhi Mu*), 9g, Radix Trichosanthis Kirlowii (*Hua Fen*), 9g, *Yu Quan San* (Jade Spring Powder)[4], 15g, wrapped during decoction, Radix Salviae Miltiorrhizae (*Dan Shen*), 15g, Radix Rubrus Paeoniae Lactiflorae (*Chi Shao*), 9g, Cortex Radicis Moutan (*Dan Pi*), 9g, Ramulus Kalopanacis Septemlobi Seu Araliae Chinensis (*Niao Bu Su*), 15g

B. Middle wasting: Stomach heat intense & exuberant

Main symptoms: Polyphagia and easy hunger, bodily emaciation, dry stool, a red tongue with a yellow coating, and a slippery, large, forceful pulse

Treatment principles: Clear the stomach and drain fire, nourish yin and quicken the blood

Rx: Rhizoma Coptidis Chinensis (*Huang Lian*), 3g, Fructus Gardeniae Jasminoidis (*Shan Zhi*), 9g, uncooked Gypsum Fibrosum (*Shi Gao*),

---

[4] This is a patent medicine composed of: Fructus Schizandrae Chinensis (*Wu Wei Zi*), Uncooked Radix Rehmanniae (*Sheng Di*), Radix Trichosanthis Kirlowii (*Tian Hua Ren*), Radix Puerariae (*Ge Gen*), and radix Glycyrrhizae (*Gan Cao*).

30g, Radix Et Rhizoma Rhei (*Da Huang*), 9g, Cortex Radicis Moutan (*Dan Pi*), 9g, Semen Pruni Persicae (*Tao Ren*), 9g, Rhizoma Phragmitis Communis (*Lu Gen*), 30g, Radix Scrophulariae Ningpoensis (*Xuan Shen*), 15g, Ramulus Kalopanacis Septemlobi Seu Aralia Chinensis (*Niao Bu Su*), 15g, Radix Scutellariae Baicalensis (*Huang Qin*), 9g

C. Lower wasting: Kidney qi deficiency & vacuity

Main symptoms: Frequent urination, amount excessive, turbid urine like fat or grease, a dry mouth, a dark, blackish complexion, scorched, dry auricles, low back and knee soreness and weakness, skin itching, impotence, premature ejaculation, a red tongue, and a fine pulse

Treatment principles: Supplement and boost the kidneys qi, nourish and quicken the blood

Rx: Tuber Ophiopogonis Japonicae (*Mai Dong*), 9g, Fructus Schizandrae Chinensis (*Wu Wei Zi*), 6g, prepared Radix Rehmanniae (*Shu Di*), 30g, Cortex Radicis Moutan (*Dan Pi*), 9g, Radix Dioscoreae Oppositae (*Shan Yao*), 15g, Sclerotium Poriae Cocos (*Fu Ling*), 9g, Fructus Corni Officinalis (*Yu Rou*), 9g, Rhizoma Alismatis (*Ze Xie*), 9g, Radix Salviae Miltiorrhizae (*Dan Shen*), 15g, Ramulus Kalopanacis Septemlobi Seu Araliae Chinensis (*Niao Bu Su*), 15g, Flos Carthami Tinctorii (*Hong Hua*), 9g

Secret Essentials

1. Large clinical strides can be made by studying wasting and thirsting based on the pathophysiology of diabetes mellitus. The pathological change associated with this disease lies in the thickening of the basal membranes in the capillary walls. Laboratory findings on the abnormal character of blood flow and on the increase in blood viscosity in this disease confirm that this disease has manifestations of stasis blood. Therefore, in treating this disease, the addition of medicinals for quickening the blood and transforming stasis is able to raise treatment efficacy.

2. Herba Euphorbiae Humifusae (*Di Jin Cao*), 30g, should be decocted and drunk as a substitute for tea. It should be taken every day. This decoction is able to decrease sugar in the urine. Its effect is particularly good in acute diabetes mellitus. If the fresh herb is used, its effects are quicker.

3. Radix Pseudostellariae (*Tai Zi Shen*), 9g, Radix Glehniae Littoralis (*Bei Sha Shen*), 10g, Gypsum Fibrosum (*Shi Gao*), 30g, Rhizoma Anemarrhenae (*Zhi Mu*), 15g, and uncooked Radix Glycyrrhizae (*Gan Cao*), 3g, should be decocted together, each day 1 *ji*. This is capable of reducing blood sugar.

6. Chronic Gastritis (*Man Xing Wei Yan*)

Chronic gastritis is categorized as stomach pain (*wei tong*) in TCM. In the *Nei Jing (Inner Classic)*, there are numerous discussions of this disease. For instance, in the chapter titled "The Forms of Diseases Caused by Evil Qi in the Viscera & Bowels" in the *Ling Shu (Spiritual Pivot)* says, "If in stomach disease, there is abdominal distension and stomach and epigastric pain which radiates upward to the lateral costal region bilaterally, the diaphragm and throat do not communicate, and food and drink to not descend, choose *Zu San Li* (St 36)." The site of the lesion, its clinical manifestations, and its treatment as described in that book are all quite similar to those of chronic gastritis. Ming Dynasty medical texts dealt definitively with the disease causes and disease mechanisms of stomach pain as well as its pattern discrimination and treatment. For instance, the *Shou Shi Bai Yuan (Protecting the Origin of Longevity)* says, "Stomach and epigastric pain is mostly due to indulging one's mouth and abdomen with a love for eating acrid and sour foods, drinking hot wine, tasting fried foods, and then eating cold, cool, or raw, chilled foods." The *Jing Yue Quan Shu (The Complete Writings of Jing-yue)* says, "The pattern of stomach and epigastric pain is mostly due to eating, cold, or qi not flowing normally." Ye Tian-shi, a famous Qing Dynasty physician, advanced his particular viewpoint that stomach pain is related to static blood. In his *Lin Zheng Zhi Nan*

(Guidebook to Clinical Patterns) in the chapter titled "Stomach & Epigastric Pain", he states:

> At first, the disease is in the channels. In enduring disease, it enters the network vessels. Because the channels govern the qi while the network vessels govern the blood, so we may know that treating the qi and blood is a matter of course. Since qi is long obstructed, the blood is also correspondingly diseased and the vessels and network vessels through which it moves will automatically be obstructed. Thus the methods of rectifying the qi with the acrid and fragrant or harmonizing blood with the acrid and softening are, in fact, absolutely necessary principles.

This theory is laden with significance in guiding clinical practice.

Disease causes, disease mechanisms

The stomach is endowed with thrusting and harmonizing qi. It should diffuse and flow freely, and it should not become depressed and stagnant. If stomach qi congests and gathers, lack of free flow leads to pain. Although stomach and epigastric pain is located in the stomach, it has close relationship with the liver. The liver pertains to wood, while the stomach pertains to earth. Wood is capable of checking earth. If one's emotions and orientation are not realized, the liver loses its orderly reaching. Qi and blood will become depressed and bound. The liver will then necessarily invade the stomach and cause aching and pain. If this endures for days, it can lead to the production of static blood. Stasis then obstructs the network vessels. The pain is like pricking. One may also see bloody stools. In addition, liver depression may transform into fire. Thus burning heat in the stomach is often seen. If there is excessive drinking and eating and irregular hunger and satiation, qi and blood will congeal, stagnate, and not flow freely, and damp heat will obstruct the center. These are also causes of this disease. Constitutional spleen and stomach vacuity weakness due to taxation and fatigue or improper use of medicinals may likewise result in damage.

Treatment based on pattern discrimination

A. Qi stagnation, blood stasis

Main symptoms: Stomach and epigastric distention and pain, fixed, stable pain which refuses pressure, chest and lateral costal glomus and fullness, burping or belching relaxes the pain, a purple tongue having static spots or patches, and a wiry, choppy pulse

Treatment principles: Course the liver and rectify the qi, quicken the blood and stop pain

Rx: Radix Salviae Miltiorrhizae (*Dan Shen*), 10 g, Lignum Santali Albi (*Tan Xiang*), 1.5g, Fructus Amomi (*Sha Ren*), 3g, Radix Saussureae Seu Vladimiriae (*Mu Xiang*), 4.5g, Rhizoma Corydalis Yanhusuo (*Yan Hu Suo*), 9g, Fructus Citri Sacrodactylis (*Fo Shou*), 4.5g, Rhizoma Cyperi Rotundi (*Xiang Fu*), 9g, Radix Linderae Strychnifoliae (*Wu Yao*), 6g, Concha Arcae (*Wa Leng Zi*), 15g, uncooked Fructus Germinatus Hordei Vulgaris (*Mai Ya*), 30g, Fructus Meliae Toosendanis (*Chuan Lian Zi*), 9g

B. Liver fire mixed with stasis

Main symptoms: Stomach and epigastric burning heat and piercing pain, very intense pain which refuses pressure, vexation and agitation, easy anger, acid eructations, a bitter taste in the mouth and dryness in the mouth, reddish urination, constipation, a purple red tongue with a yellow coating, and a wiry, rapid pulse

Treatment principles: Course the liver and discharge fire, quicken the blood and stop pain

Rx: Cortex Radicis Moutan (*Dan Pi*), 9g, Fructus Gardeniae Jasminoidis (*Shan Zhi*), 9g, Pericarpium Viridis Citri Reticulatae (*Qing Pi*), 4.5g, Pericarpium Citri Reticulatae (*Chen Pi*), 4.5g, Radix Albus

Paeoniae Lactiflorae (*Bai Shao*), 9g, Bulbus Fritillariae Thunbergii (*Xiang Bei*), 9g, Rhizoma Corydalis Yanhusuo (*Yan Hu Suo*), 9g, Fructus Meliae Toosendanis (*Chuan Lian Zi*), 9g, Radix Glycyrrhizae (*Gan Cao*), 3g, Herba Cum Radice Taraxaci Mongolici (*Pu Gong Ying*), 15g, *Zuo Jin Wan* (Left Gold Pills)[5], 4.5g, Aspongopus (*Jiu Xiang Chong*), 2.4g

C. Phlegm & stasis binding together

Main symptoms: Stomach and epigastric pricking pain, enduring pain which does not heal, immovable pain, pain mild in the day and severe at night, chest oppression, excessive phlegm, dry throat, turbid qi (*i.e.*, foul-smelling flatulence), a dark, purple tongue with a thick, slimy coating, and a wiry, slippery pulse

Treatment principles: Quicken the blood and open the network vessels, transform phlegm and harmonize the stomach

Rx: Caulis In Taeniis Bambusae (*Zhu Ru*), 6g, Fructus Citri Seu Ponciri (*Zhi Qiao*), 9g, Pericarpium Viridis Citri Reticulatae (*Qing Pi*), 4.5g, Pericarpium Citri Reticulatae (*Chen Pi*), 4.5g, Sclerotium Poriae Cocos (*Fu Ling*), 9g, Rhizoma Pinelliae Ternatae (*Ban Xia*), 9g, uncooked Pollen Typhae (*Pu Huang*), 9g, wrapped during decoction, Concha Arcae (*Wa Leng Zi*), 9g, clear, mix-fried Radix Glycyrrhizae (*Zhi Gan Cao*), 3g, Fructus Piperis Cubebae (*Bi Cheng Qie*), 4.5g, Haematitum (*Dai Zhe Shi*), 30g, Fructus Piperis Longi (*Bi Ba*), 3g

D. Cold & stasis congealing and binding

Main symptoms: Stomach and epigastric intense, colicky pain, fear of cold by the affected area, relaxation when it obtains warmth, poor

---

[5] This is a patent medicine composed of: Ginger(-processed) Rhizoma Coptidis Chinensis (*Huang Lian*) and Fructus Evodiae Rutecarpae (*Wu Zhu Yu*).

appetite, loose stool, a pale, purple tongue with thin, white coating, and a wiry, tight pulse

Treatment principles: Quicken the blood and open the network vessels, dispel cold and stop pain

Rx: Radix Lateralis Praeparatus Aconiti Carmichaeli (*Dan Fu Pian*), 6g, vinegar(-processed) Feces Trogopterori Seu Pteromi (*Ling Zhi*), 9g, Fructus Meliae Toosendanis (*Chuan Lian Zi*), 9g, Fructus Foeniculi Vulgaris (*Xiao Hui Xiang*), 4.5g, Rhizoma Alpiniae Officinari (*Gao Liang Jiang*), 4.5g, Rhizoma Cyperi Rotundi (*Xiang Fu*), 9g, Rhizoma Atractylodis Macrocephalae (*Bai Zhu*), 9g, Fructus Citri Seu Ponciri (*Zhi Qiao*), 9g, Cortex Cinnamomi (*Rou Gui*), 1.5g, Fructus Evodiae Rutecarpae (*Wu Zhu Yu*), 2.4g, Rhizoma Corydalis Yanhusuo (*Yan Hu Suo*), 9g

Secret Essentials

1. In treating this disease, first regulate and disinhibit the qi mechanism. Secondly, quicken the blood and transform stasis. The following is the great method of using medicinals: For qi repletion, rectify it. Commonly used medicinals are Pericarpium Viridis Citri Reticulatae (*Qing Pi*), Pericarpium Citri Reticulatae (*Chen Pi*), Pericarpium Citri Medicare (*Xiang Yuan Pi*), Fructus Citri Sarcodactylis (*Fo Shou*), Rhizoma Cyperi Rotundi (*Xiang Fu*), Radix Saussureae Seu Vladimiriae (*Mu Xiang*), Tuber Curcumae (*Yu Jin*), and Lignum Aquilariae Agallochae (*Chen Xiang*). For blood repletion, sequence it. It is all right to first use Radix Salviae Miltiorrhizae (*Dan Shen*), Radix Rubrus Paeoniae Lactiflorae (*Chi Shao*), Semen Pruni Persicae (*Tao Ren*), Flos Carthami Tinctorii (*Hong Hua*), Rhizoma Corydalis Yanhusuo (*Yan Hu Suo*), Feces Trogopterori Seu Pteromi (*Wu Ling Zhi*), and Radix Angelicae Sinensis (*Dang Gui*). If the stools are mixed with occult blood, add equal portions of powdered Radix Pseudoginseng (*San Qi*), Rhizoma Bletillae Striatae (*Bai Ji*), and Pollen Typhae (*Pu Huang*). Take 3g each time, 3 times per day. If the pain radiates to the lateral costal region bilaterally, then it is all right to add Radix Bupleuri (*Chai Hu*) and

Concha Arcae (*Wa Leng Zi*). If stomach yin is damaged, add Radix Glehniae Littoralis (*Sha Shen*), Rhizoma Polygonati Odorati (*Yu Zhu*), Semen Dolichoris Lablabis (*Bian Dou*), and uncooked Fructus Germinatus Hordei (*Mai Ya*). If gastroscopic examination shows that the mucous membranes in the stomach are bright red, then stasis heat is obstructing internally, Correspondingly add Herba Cum Radice Taraxaci Mongolici (*Pu Gong Ying*) or Herba Oldenlandiae Diffusae (*Bai Hua She She Cao*). For atrophic gastritis, add Fructus Pruni Mume (*Wu Mei*), 9-15g.

2. Stomach pain has a close relationship with liver depression. If the disease is enduring, the heart mind will be worried and depressed. Correspondingly, one should take care to regulate and disinhibit the liver qi. Therefore, I like to add to formulas for this condition Fructus Akebiae Trifoliatae (*Ba Yue Zha*), Fructus Aesculi (*Suo Luo Zi*), and Flos Pruni Mume (*Lu O Mei*). In addition, medicinal cakes are also important since they can cheer up the emotions and nourish one's disposition.

7. Female Climacteric Syndrome (*Nu Xing Geng Nian Qi Zong He Zheng*)

The climacteric is the turning point from maturity to decline in female physiological function. Thus it may also be seen as a transitional stage before entering the period of senility. Beginning from 45 years of age or so, ovarian function gradually declines until at last it disappears altogether. After menopause, progressive degeneration in tissue occurs, gradually causing decline and senility. These changes in the internal environment lead to a series of endocrine functional disturbances as well as to symptoms of dysfunction in the autonomic nervous system. These symptoms are different in individual patients due to differences in constitution and the environment in which they live. In particular, these symptoms have a close relationship with the patients' essence spirit (*i.e.*, mental/emotional) factors. Typical symptoms include vexation and agitation, worry, depression, and anxiety. These are categorized as depression pattern (*yu zheng*), visceral agitation (*zang zao*), and lily disease (*bai he bing*) in our national medicine (*i.e.*, TCM). Mostly, these symptoms occur just before or after menopause.

Disease causes, disease mechanisms

Before menopause, a woman's visceral qi has already become thin (*i.e.*, weak). This is the internal factor for the occurrence of this disease. Emotional factors, the degree of strength of stimulation of the essence spirit, and their duration are interrelated and are even more closely related to the condition of the organism. The constructive and defensive gradually decline. Heart qi is insufficient. The liver loses its regulation and reaching. Kidney essence is deficient and vacuous. The brain loses its nourishment. The spirit brilliance has nothing on which to depend. Qi and blood are perverse and disobedient. The essence spirit is absent-minded. And symptoms gradually proceed from a mild to a serious condition. Vacuity and repletion appear together.

Treatment based on pattern discrimination

A. Heart spirit bewildered & chaotic

Main symptoms: The mental state is not calm. The heart spirit is abstracted. Sadness is so damaging one feels like weeping. The form and spirit are tired and fatigued. There is scant qi, disinclination to speak, frequent yawning, spontaneous perspiration, chilled limbs, poor appetite and no taste, diarrhea, loose stools, a pale tongue with a white coating, and a deep, fine, and weak pulse

Treatment principles: Supplement the qi and boost yang, quicken the blood and transform stasis

Rx: Radix Lateralis Praeparatus Aconiti Carmichaeli (*Fu Pian*), 9g, Os Draconis (*Long Gu*), 30g, Concha Ostreae (*Mu Li*), 30g, Ramulus Cinnamomi (*Gui Zhi*), 4.5g, Radix Albus Paeoniae Lactiflorae (*Bai Shao*), 9g, mix-fried Radix Polygalae Tenuifoliae (*Yuan Zhi*), 9g, Semen Ziziphi Spinosae (*Zao Ren*), 9g, Rhizoma Atractylodis Macrocephalae (*Bai Zhu*), 9g, Radix Salviae Miltiorrhizae (*Dan Shen*), 15g, Radix Bupleuri (*Chai Hu*), 9g, Flos Carthami Tinctorii (*Hong Hua*), 9g

B. Heart blood deficiency & vacuity

Main symptoms: Heart palpitations, restlessness, heart vexation, scant sleep, excessive suspicion, easy anger, nervous tension, apprehension, anxiety, a dry mouth, a bitter taste in the mouth, night fever, and vexation and agitation, red urine, constipation, a red tongue, and a rapid pulse

Treatment principles: Nourish the blood and calm the heart, quicken the blood and transform stasis

Rx: Mix-fried Radix Glycyrrhizae (*Zhi Gan Cao*), 4.5g, Fructus Levis Tritici (*Huai Xiao Mai*), 30g, Fructus Zizyphi Jujubae (*Hong Zao*), 5 pieces, Radix Polygalae Tenuifoliae (*Yuan Zhi*), 9g, Sclerotium Pararadicis Poriae Cocos (*Fu Shen*), 9g, Radix Salviae Miltiorrhizae (*Dan Shen*), 15g, Bulbus Lilii (*Bai He*), 9g, Plumula Nelumbinis Nuciferae (*Lian Zi Xin*), 4.5g, Rhizoma Anemarrhenae (*Zhi Mu*), 9g, Radix Angelicae Sinensis (*Dang Gui*), 9g, Radix Ligustici Wallichii (*Chuan Xiong*), 4.5g, Semen Ziziphi Spinosae (*Zao Ren*), 9g

C. Liver qi depression & binding

Main symptoms: Essence spirit worry and depression, nervous tension, apprehension, chest oppression, heaving sighs, sometimes cold, sometimes hot, dizziness, vexation and agitation, lateral costal distention and pain, epigastric and abdominal discomfort, easy anger, easy fright, a red face and eyes, a bluish tongue with a dry coating, and a wiry, rapid pulse

Treatment principles: Soothe the liver and resolve depression, quicken the blood and transform stasis

Rx: Cortex Radicis Moutan (*Dan Pi*), 9g, Fructus Gardeniae Jasminoidis (*Shan Zhi*), 9g, Herba Menthae Haplocalycis (*Bo He*), 4.5g, Rhizoma Acori Graminei (*Chang Pu*), 4.5g, Radix Ligustici Wallichii (*Chuan Xiong*), 4.5g, Semen Pruni Persicae (*Tao Ren*), 9g, Radix Rubrus Paeoniae Lactiflorae (*Chi Shao*), 9g, Radix Bupleuri (*Chai Hu*), 9g, Fructus Citri Seu Ponciri (*Zhi Qiao*), 6g, Radix Platycodi Grandiflori (*Jie Geng*), 6g, Radix Angelicae Sinensis (*Dang Gui*), 9g, powdered Margarita (*Zhen Zhu*), 1g, powdered Succinum (*Hu Po*), 1g, these last two powders to be washed down by the other decocted medicinals

8. Male Climacteric Syndrome (*Nan Xing Geng Nian Qi Zong He Zheng*)

Climacteric syndrome in males generally occurs after 55 years of age, somewhat later than it does in females. Influenced by such factors as constitution, lifestyle, and mental state, this syndrome may occur earlier or later. Owing to gradual degeneration of the testicles leading to imbalance in viscera and bowel function, it is characterized clinically by obesity and change in temperament. In severe cases, it may affect one's work and life activities.

Disease causes, disease mechanisms

Climacteric syndrome occurs after the fifth decade when the organism can no longer carry on its self-regulation or maintain the relative balance between yin and yang. Its main pattern is kidney yin deficiency and vacuity. However, there may also occur various patterns where kidney yang deficiency and vacuity or both kidney yin and kidney yang deficiency may be seen. Essence spirit factors are the external causes of the onset of this disease.

Treatment based on pattern discrimination

A. Yin vacuity, internal heat

Main symptoms: Tidal fever, night sweats, vertigo and dizziness, tinnitus, an uneasy feeling in the eyes and fear of light, blurred vision, diminished force of memory, tension and agitation, decline in sexual function or premature ejaculation, a red tongue with a thin coating, and a fine, rapid pulse

Treatment principles: Enrich and supplement kidney yin, clear heat and quicken the blood

Rx: Rhizoma Anemarrhenae (*Zhi Mu*), 9g, Cortex Phellodendri (*Huang Bai*), 9g, uncooked Radix Rehmanniae (*Sheng Di*), 15g, Cortex Radicis Moutan (*Dan Pi*), 9g, Rhizoma Alismatis (*Ze Xie*), 9g, Radix Dioscoreae Oppositae (*Shan Yao*), 15g, Sclerotium Poriae Cocos (*Fu Ling*), 9g, mix-fried Carapax Amydae Sinensis (*Bie Jia*), 15g, mix-fried Plastrum Testudinis (*Gui Ban*), 15g, calcined Concha Ostreae (*Mu Li*), 30g, Fructus Corni Officinalis (*Yu Rou*), 9g, Semen Pruni Persicae (*Tao Ren*), 9g

B. Kidney yin & yang dual vacuity

Main symptoms: Dizziness, tinnitus, loss of sleep, poor memory, lack of constancy in joy and anger, sudden feelings of heat, sweating, fear of cold, dread of chill, a bright white complexion, shortness of breath, low back and knee soreness and weakness, superficial edema, loose stools, decline in sexual function, a pale tongue with a thin coating, and a fine, weak pulse

Treatment principles: Supplement both yin and yang, quicken the blood and transform stasis

Rx: Rhizoma Curculiginis Orchoidis (*Xian Mao*), 9g, Herba Epimedii (*Xian Ling Pi*), 9g, Radix Morindae Officinalis (*Ba Ji Tian*), 9g, Herba Cistanchis (*Rou Cong Rong*), 9g, Fructus Lycii Chinensis (*Qi Zi*), 9g, Semen Cuscutae (*Tu Si Zi*), 9g, Radix Angelicae Sinensis (*Dang Gui*), 9g, Radix Achyranthis Bidentatae (*Niu Xi*), 9g, Cornu Cervi (*Lu Jiao*), 9g, Radix Salviae Miltiorrhizae (*Dan Shen*), 15g

C. Liver qi depression & binding

Main symptoms: Essence spirit depression, emotional unease, chest fullness and oppression, lateral costal and distention and pain, easy agitation, easy anger, epigastric oppression, belching, no thought for eating and drinking, irregular defecation, a thin tongue coating, and a wiry pulse

Treatment principles: Course the liver and resolve depression, nourish and quicken the blood

Rx: Radix Bupleuri (*Chai Hu*), 6g, Cortex Radicis Moutan (*Dan Pi*), 9g, Radix Ligustici Wallichii (*Chuan Xiong*), 4.5g, Radix Rubrus Paeoniae Lactiflorae (*Chi Shao*), 9g, Rhizoma Cyperi Rotundi (*Xiang Fu*), 9g, Radix Salviae Miltiorrhizae (*Dan Shen*), 15g, Tuber Curcumae (*Yu Jin*), 9g, Radix Angelicae Sinensis (*Dang Gui*), 9g, Ramulus Uncariae Cum Uncis (*Shuang Gou*), 9g, Fructus Akebiae Trifoliatae (*Ba Yue Zha*), 9g, Semen Aesculi (*Suo Luo Zi*), 9g, Flos Pruni Mume (*Lu O Mei*), 4.5g

Secret Essentials (for both male and female climacteric syndrome)

1. The climacteric is a normal physiological stage. If one is able to correctly and calmly deal with its symptoms without worry, fear, agitation, or anger, then, after a certain period, the endocrine system will re-establish its balance and the symptoms will spontaneously disappear. In other words, psychological balance can help improve of this disease's symptoms.

2. One should also do proper physical training to improve and raise their body and corporeal soul. They should take care to regulate and discipline drinking and diet, and eat less sweet, fatty, thick flavored foods but more vegetables and fruits so that their body may avoid becoming over-weight.

3. One should keep their genitalia clean. This is because, after one enters the climacteric, the mucous membranes in the genitals becomes thin and frail and topical resistance is weakened. Therefore, the region may easily become infected.

4. If it is difficult for one to eliminate emotional depression, then *Xue Fu Zhu Yu Tang* (Blood Mansion Dispel Stasis Decoction) is all right to use to regulate and put in good order yin and yang and to balance qi and blood: Radix Bupleuri (*Chai Hu*), 4.5g, Radix Ligustici Wallichii (*Chuan Xiong*), 4.5g, Radix Angelicae Sinensis (*Dang Gui*), 9g, Flos Carthami Tinctorii (*Hong Hua*), 9g, Radix Rubrus Paeoniae Lactiflorae (*Chi Shao*), 9g, uncooked Radix Rehmanniae (*Sheng Di*), 12g, Radix Glycyrrhizae (*Gan Cao*), 3g, Fructus Citri Seu Ponciri (*Zhi Qiao*), 4.5g, Radix Platycodi Grandiflori (*Jie Geng*), 4.5g, Radix Achyranthis Bidentatae (*Niu Xi*), 4.5g, Semen Pruni Persicae (*Tao Ren*), 9g. This may encourage one's emotions and stimulate one's essence spirit. All emotional diseases should be treated based on the blood aspect. Clinically, this is very valuable.

9. Scleroderma (*Ying Pi Bing*)

Scleroderma is a kind of slowly progressive disease whose etiology is still not clearly understood. It is characterized by fibrosis or sclerosis and finally atrophy of localized or diffuse skin and connective tissues in the internal organs. This disease corresponds to skin *bi* in our national medicine (*i.e.*, TCM). Owing to qi and blood stasis and stagnation, the skin gradually becomes scaly and dry, eventually becoming like horn. This may also eventually affect the internal organs. Engenderment and transformation lose their normalcy, and the patient's life destiny may be endangered. This is categorized as a difficult to treat disease.

Disease causes, disease mechanisms

Initially, the lungs and kidneys are vacuous and suffer detriment. The defensive outside is not secure and the interstices lose their dense packing. Secondarily, wind, cold, and damp evils invade the body, resulting in constructive blood not being full. Blood movement is inhibited, and cold congeals, astringes, and stagnates. This adds to and aggravates obstruction and stasis of the blood vessels. The interstices lose their nourishment and thus the skin becomes hard.

Treatment based on pattern discrimination

The internal cause of this disease is lung/kidney yang vacuity, while the external cause is wind, cold, damp evils. When the qi and blood in the channels and network vessels obtain heat, they become moist. If they meet with cold, they become congealed or astringed. Therefore, the general treatment principle is to adopt simultaneously the two methods of warming yang and opening *bi* and quickening the blood and transforming stasis.

Main symptoms: The face, hands, feet, and even the skin of the whole body gradually become sclerotic with a shiny color and visible deep pigmentation.

Treatment principles: Warm yang and open *bi*, quicken the blood and transform stasis

Rx: Rhizoma Sparganii (*San Leng*), 9g, Rhizoma Curcumae Zedoariae (*E Zhu*), 9g, Radix Astragali Membranacei (*Huang Qi*), 30g, Herba Ephedrae (*Ma Huang*), 10g, Hirudo (*Shui Zhi*), 3g, Radix Clematidis Chinensis (*Wei Ling Xian*), 9g, Flos Carthami Tinctorii (*Hong Hua*), 9g, Radix Rubrus Paeoniae Lactiflorae (*Chi Shao*), 12g, Radix Ligustici Wallichii (*Chuan Xiong*), 9g, Herba Sargassii (*Hai Zao*), 9g, Thallus Algae (*Kun Bu*), 9g, uncooked Concha Ostreae (*Mu Li*), 30g, Radix Lateralis Praeparatus Aconiti Carmichaeli (*Fu Pian*), 6g

Secret Essentials

1. The treatment of this disease should correspond to first opening yang, boosting the qi, and transforming stasis. If the above formula is not effective, it is all right to choose *Tong Mai Si Ni Tang* (Open the Vessels Four Counterflows Decoction): mix-fried Radix Glycyrrhizae (*Zhi Gan Cao*), 4.5g, Radix Lateralis Praeparatus Aconiti Carmichaeli (*Fu Zi*), 15g, dry Rhizoma Zingiberis (*Gan Jiang*), 2.4g, Bulbus Allii Fistulosi (*Cong*), 5 stalks, plus Ramulus Cinnamomi (*Gui Zhi*), 6g, Radix Rubrus Paeoniae Lactiflorae (*Chi Shao*), 9g, Semen Pruni Persicae (*Tao Ren*), 9g, and Hirudo (*Shui Zhi*), 3g, in order to warm yang and transform congelation.

2. In treating this disease, one should pay attention to the method of diffusing the lungs, since the lungs govern the skin and hair. In mild cases, Radix Asteris Tatarici (*Zi Wan*) should be used. In severe case, Herba Ephedrae (*Ma Huang*) may be selected. The dosage should be heavy. The dose I frequently use is more than 10g.

3. For localized scleroderma, it is all right to use three decoctions of the above formula mixed with 1 cupful of white alcohol (*Bai Jiu*) as an external wash of the affected area. Continue until it becomes red.

4. Wang Qing-ren's *Tong Qiao Huo Xue Tang* (Open the Portals & Quicken Blood Decoction) is also effective: Radix Rubrus Paeoniae Lactiflorae (*Chi Shao*), 9g, Radix Ligustici Wallichii (*Chuan Xiong*), 9g, Semen Pruni Persicae (*Tao Ren*), 9g, Flos Carthami Tinctorii (*Hong Hua*), 9g, Secretio Moschi Moschiferi (*She Xiang*), 0.3g, old Bulbus Allii Fistulosi (*Lao Cong*), 5 stalks.

10. Herpes Zoster (*Dai Zhuang Pao Zhen*)

Herpes zoster causes water blisters. It is caused by the herpes zoster virus. At first there occur red patches. On these red patches there then appear groups of pearl-like water blisters. In the center of these vesicles, there is a sort of umbilicus which contains blood blisters and pus blisters. Groups of water blisters are distributed along the nerves. The virus lies dormant in the spinal root ganglia or in the trigeminal nerve ganglia. The disease erupts when the immunity of the organism is lowered. If the posterior root of the foot spinal nerve is involved, it may cause intense aching and pain. The older the patient, the more severe will this aching and pain be. Even after the eruption of water blisters subsides completely, aching and pain may persist for from several months to half a year. Because this eruption is prone to occur around the waist, in TCM it is called low back girdling fire cinnabar (*chan yao huo dan*). In addition, because the vesicular rash is shaped like a snake, it is also called snake cinnabar (*she dan*).

Disease causes, disease mechanisms

The *Wai Ke Zheng Zong (Orthodox Ancestral External Medicine)* states that, in terms of this disease:

> Heart fire recklessly stirs. Wind heat in the three warmers takes advantage of this and causes eruption on the skin.

The eruption of the vesicles may also be due to emotions and orientation causing internal damage with depressive liver/gallbladder fire accumulating; spleen dampness smoldering internally; and external contraction of toxic evils. Toxic evils, depressive fire, and damp heat struggle and bind, obstructing the channels and network vessels. Hence qi and blood do not flow freely and this disease results.

Treatment based on pattern discrimination

A. Liver/gallbladder depressive fire

Main symptoms: Herpes lesions which are tidal red, spots and dots like millet which gather into patches, burning heat, aching and pain, a red tongue with a yellow coating, and a wiry, rapid pulse

Treatment principles: Clear the liver and drain fire, quicken the blood and transform toxins

Rx: Radix Gentianae Scabrae (*Long Dan Cao*), 9g, Rhizoma Coptidis Chinensis (*Huang Lian*), 3g, Radix Scutellariae Baicalensis (*Huang Qin*), 9g, Cortex Radicis Moutan (*Dan Pi*), 9g, Radix Rubrus Paeoniae Lactiflorae (*Chi Shao*), 9g, Radix Lithopsermi Seu Arnebiae (*Zi Cao*), 9g, Flos Chrysanthemi Morifolii (*Ju Hua*), 9g, Flos Lonicerae Japonicae (*Yin Hua*), 9g, Folium Isatidis (*Da Qing Ye*), 15g, uncooked Radix Rehmanniae (*Sheng Di*), 15g, Semen Pruni Persicae (*Tao Ren*), 9g

B. Spleen dampness internally smoldering

Main symptoms: In the skin there arises yellowish white blisters filled with turbid fluid. They easily break and the fluid flows out. The aching and pain then become particularly acute. In addition, there is torpid intake, abdominal distention, and soy sauce-like stools. The pulse is slippery and rapid, and the tongue coating is white and slimy.

Treatment principles: Clear and disinhibit dampness and heat, quicken the blood and transform toxins

Rx: Rhizoma Atractylodis (*Cang Zhu*), 9g, Rhizoma Atractylodis Macrocephalae (*Bai Zhu*), 9g, Cortex Phellodendri (*Huang Bai*), 9g, Radix Achyranthis Bidentatae (*Niu Xi*), 9g, Rhizoma Smilacis Glabrae (*Tu Fu Ling*), 30g, Herba Leonuri Heterophylli (*Yi Mu Cao*), 30g, *Liu Yi San* (Six to One Powder)[6], 9g, wrapped during decoction, Rhizoma Dioscoreae Hypoglaucae (*Fen Bi Xie*), 9g, Cortex Radicis Moutan (*Dan Pi*), 9g, Radix Lithospermi Seu Arnebiae (*Zi Cao*), 9g, uncooked Semen Coicis Lachryma-jobi (*Mi Ren*), 30g, Radix Isatidis Seu Baphicacanthi (*Ban Lan Gen*), 30g

---

[6] This refers to a mixture of 6 parts Talcum (*Hua Shi*) to 1 part Radix Glycyrrhizae (*Gan Cao*).

C. Blood stasis & qi stagnation

Main symptoms: The base of the herpes lesions are dark and purple. The fluid contains bloody water. Aching and pain is acute and difficult to bear. The tongue is purple and dark or has static patches. The pulse is wiry and choppy.

Treatment principles: Quicken the blood and transform toxins, move the qi and stop pain

Rx: Uncooked Radix Rehmanniae (*Sheng Di*), 15g, Hirudo (*Shui Zhi*), 3g, Guangdong Lumbricus (*Guang Di Long*), 9g, uncooked Semen Coicis Lachryma-jobi (*Mi Ren*), 30g, Radix Rubrus Paeoniae Lacti-florae (*Chi Shao*), 9g, Cortex Radicis Moutan (*Dan Pi*), 9g, uncooked Pollen Typhae (*Pu Huang*), 9g, wrapped during decoction, Radix Salviae Miltiorrhizae (*Dan Shen*), 15g, Rhizoma Smilacis Glabrae (*Tu Fu Ling*), 30g, Herba Portulacae Oleraceae (*Ma Chi Xian*), 30g

Secret Essentials

1. This disease is categorized as qi and blood congestion and obstruction by evil toxins. Qi is stagnant and blood is static. Internally, there is excessive depressive heat. Therefore, there are mouth prohibitions regarding eating and drinking.[7] Smoking, alcohol, and acrid, peppery food are not appropriate.

2. If the disease has persisted and is not cured, the righteous qi has already declined, and stasis heat has consumed yin, it is all right to use *Liu Wei Di Huang Wan* (Six Flavors Rehmannia Pills)[8] to support the

---

[7] Mouth prohibitions means prohibition regarding certain foods and drinks.

[8] These are composed of Prepared Radix Rehmanniae (*Shu Di*), Radix Dioscoreae Oppositate (*Shan Yao*), Fructus Corni Officinalis (*Shan Zhu Yu*), Sclerotium Poriae Cocos (*Fu Ling*), Rhizoma Alismatis (*Ze Xie*), and Cortex Radicis Moutan (*Dan Pi*).

righteous qi and eliminate evils. Take 9g each time, 2 times per day.

3. Realgar (*Xiong Huang*), 9g, mixed with glycerin, may be applied externally on the affected area 2-3 times per day.

4. Acupuncture: Needle *Nei Guan* (Per 6) through to *Wai Guan* (TH 5) and *Qui Xu* (GB 40) through to *Zhao Hai* (Ki 6), once every other day. Or one may use *Dang Gui Zhu Ze Ye* (Dang Gui Injectible Fluid) injected into *Fei Shu* (Bl 13), 2ml each time, 1 time per day.

11. Senile Pruritus

Pruritus is a commonly seen geriatric disease. It is caused by dryness of the skin, degenerative atrophy, and decline in the function of sebaceous and sweat glands. However, arteriosclerosis in the nervous system or allergens in certain substances are also important disease causes.

Disease causes, disease mechanisms

In TCM it is said that, "Pain, sores, and itching all pertain to the heart." The heart governs the blood. Therefore, itching pertains to either blood heat or blood vacuity. It is also said that, "All itching pertains to wind." Eliminating external affection by the wind evils, blood vacuity can also engender wind. Senile pruritus is mostly categorized as blood vacuity engendering wind or blood heat mixed with external wind.

Treatment based on pattern discrimination

Main symptoms: At first, itching is confined to a certain spot. Later it spreads to the whole body. Pruritus may occur episodically. Traces of scratching may be seen on the skin, bloody scabs, deep pigmentation, or changes due to lichenification. These are liable to occur around the genitalia where dampness, chapping, and thickening of skin may often be observed. There is a red tongue with a white coating as well as a floating, rapid pulse.

Treatment principles: Nourish and quicken the blood, dispel wind and stop itching

Rx: Radix Angelicae Sinensis (*Dang Gui*), 9g, Rhizoma Polygonati Odorati (*Yu Zhu*), 9g, Fructus Ligustri Lucidi (*Nu Zhen Zi*), 9g, Cortex Radicis Moutan (*Dan Pi*), 9g, Radix Rubrus Paeoniae Lactiflorae (*Chi Shao*), 9g, uncooked Radix Rehmanniae (*Sheng Di*), 12 g, Cortex Radicis Lycii (*Di Gu Pi*), 9g, Herba Lemnae Seu Spirodelae (*Fu Ping*), 9g, Fructus Xanthii (*Cang Er Zi*), 9g, Cortex Radicis Dictamni (*Bai Xian Pi*), 9g, black Semen Sesami Indici (*Hei Zhi Ma*), 9g

Secret Essentials

1. One should protect one's essence spirit cheerfulness and avoid overstrain, emotional tension, worry, and anxiety. The fire of the five orientations consumes and damages blood and fluids. Blood vacuity engendering wind exacerbates pruritus, while stewing and boiling transform (*i.e.*, engender) stasis and exacerbate the pain.

2. One should protect the cleanliness of one's skin. In taking a bath, the water one uses should not be too hot. Nor should one use alkaline soap or wear clothes made from synthetic fibers.

3. One should abstain from smoking, alcohol, irritating foods, and allergenic things, such as old chicken, seafood, and mutton. They should keep their bowels open and uninhibited in order to excrete metabolic waste products.

4. Take regularly *Sang Ma Wan* (Morus & Ephedra Pills)[9], 9g each time, 2 times per day. The flavor (*i.e.*, the medicinal) Rhizoma Polygonatae Odorati (*Yu Zhu*) steamed in water may be used to rub the body after bathing. These two methods can both moisten the skin and muscles, dispel wind, and stop itching.

12. Chronic Hepatitis & Cirrhosis of the Liver (*Man Xing Gan Yan He Gan Ying Hua*)

Chronic hepatitis refers to liver inflammation persisting over 6 months and caused by a virus, medicine, or other factors. Liver cirrhosis is a chronic, systemic disease chiefly characterized by degenerative necrosis of the liver cells and destruction of the structure and proliferation of fibrous tissue. It is mostly caused by chronic hepatitis, schistosomiasis, chronic nutritional deficiency, and chronic alcoholism. Chronic hepatitis and liver cirrhosis are often lingering and cannot be cured. Cirrhosis at its terminal stage is often complicated by hepatic coma and hemorrhage of the upper digestive tract. It may also transform into liver cancer.

In TCM, chronic hepatitis and liver cirrhosis are categorized as lateral costal pain (*xie tong*), drum distention (*gu zhang*), and concretions and conglomerations (*zheng jia*), and these are closely related to qi stagnation and blood stasis. The chapter titled "The Five Evils" in the *Ling Shu (Spiritual Pivot)* says, "When evils are located in the liver, then there will be pain in the two lateral costal regions .... for there is malign blood internally." The *Mai Yi Zheng Zhi (The Treatment of Patterns Based on the Pulse)* says, "If static blood, malign blood stops and is retained in the liver, it extends below the lateral costal region and there is pain." If the disease develops into drum distention or concretions and

---

[9] These pills are comprised of: Folijm Mori Albi (*Sang Ye*), 300 g, and black Semen Sesami Indici (*Hei Zhi Ma*), 120 g. A concentrate is made from the Sesame Seeds and this and athe powdered first medicinal are added to 300 g of honey and made into 9g pills.

conglomerations, it is categorized as a difficult-to-treat disease. In ancient times, there was the saying that "wind, taxation, drum (distention), and diaphragmatic (obstruction)" are the four great difficult-to-treat diseases. However, if the disease is discovered in its early stage and treated in time and if the patient is disciplined in eating and drinking and has a regular lifestyle, then one can get a certain therapeutic effect.

Disease causes, disease mechanisms

Hepatitis means that damp heat has invaded the liver and gallbladder. The liver and gallbladder's mechanism of coursing and discharging is thus scanty. The liver is located below the lateral costal region, while the gallbladder is attached between the lobes of the liver. Once invaded by evils, the liver qi becomes depressed and bound. If this endures, it will become chronic. Qi disease will extend to the blood, while stasis will congeal in the liver network vessels. This results in hinderance and lack of free flow. The disease mechanism of drum distention lies in qi binding, blood congelation, and fluid stoppage. The disease causes are mostly damage by food and drink, emotions and orientation not being fulfilled, taxation beyond limit, and lack of treatment of chronic hepatitis. Drum distention involves the three viscera, the liver, spleen, and kidneys. It is like chronic hepatitis which is a disease in the same viscera and bowels. When the disease develops into drum distention, evils have gathered in the viscera. The former disease is relatively mild, while the latter is recalcitrant.

Treatment based on pattern discrimination

A. Dampness causing blood stasis

Main symptoms: Bilateral insidious pain in the lateral costal regions made worse by pressure. epigastric and abdominl distention and oppression, devitalized appetite, loose stools, short, sacnty urination, a pale, purple tongue with a slimy coating, and a wiry, choppy pulse

Treatment principles: Fortify the spleen and dispel dampness, quicken the blood and transform stasis

Rx: Rhizoma Atractylodis (*Cang Zhu*), 9g, Rhizoma Atractylodis Macrocephalae (*Bai Zhu*), 9g, Sclerotium Poriae Cocos (*Fu Ling*), 9g, Cortex Magnoliae Officinalis (*Chuan Po*), 6g, Pericarpium Viridis Citri Reticulatae (*Qing Pi*), 4.5g, Pericarpium Citri Reticulatae (*Chen Pi*), 4.5g, Radix Saussureae Seu Vladimiriae (*Mu Xiang*), 4.5g, Sichuan Rhizoma Coptidis Chinensis (*Chuan Lian*), 2.4g, Radix Salviae Miltiorrhizae (*Dan Shen*), 15g, Radix Rubrus Paeoniae Lactiflorae (*Chi Shao*), 9g, scorched Crataegus Massa Medica Fermentata (*Zha Qu*), 9g, Radix Ligustici Wallichii (*Chuan Xiong*), 6g, Radix Bupleuri (*Chai Hu*), 6g, *Shi Xiao San* (Sudden Smile Powder), 9g

B. Damp heat mixed with stasis

Main symptoms: Lateral costal burning heat and aching and pain, chest and epigastric bitterness and fullness, enlarged, distended abdomen, vexatious heat, oral thirst but no desire to drink rinsing water, red, astringent urination, constipation or loose stools like rotten soy sauce, a purple red tongue with a grayish yellow coating, and a wiry, rapid pulse

Treatment principles: Clear heat and disinhibit dampness, cool the constructive and quicken the blood

Rx: Powdered Cornu Bubali (*Guang Jiao*), 3g, washed down with the other decocted medicinals, Herba Lycopi Lucidi (*Ze Lan*), 15g, Rhizoma Atractylodis (*Cang Zhu*), 9g, Herba Ardisiae Japonicae (*Ping Di Mu*), 30g, Herba Lysimachiae Christinae (*Xian Ren Dui Zuo Cao*), 30g, Rhizoma Smilacis Glabrae (*Tu Fu Ling*), 15g, Radix Et Rhizoma Rhei (*Da Huang*), 9g, Cortex Radicis Moutan (*Dan Pi*), 9g, Herba Patriniae Heterophyllae (*Bai Jiang Cao*), 15g

C. Liver blood stasis & obstruction

Main symptoms: A dark complexion, lateral costal oppression, distention, and piercing pain, feeling of a concretion, conglomeration, accumulation, or lump on palpation of the abdomen, distended and engorged vessels on the abdominal wall, scaly skin, a static, purple tongue, and a deep and wiry or wiry and choppy pulse

Treatment principles: Quicken the blood and transform stasis, soften the hard and open the network vessels

Rx: Radix Et Rhizoma Rhei (*Da Huang*), 9g, Semen Pruni Persicae (*Tao Ren*), 9g, Eupolyphaga Seu Ophisthoplatia (*Di Bie Zhong*), 4.5g, Radix Salviae Miltiorrhizae (*Dan Shen*), 15g, Radix Ligustici Wallichii (*Chuan Xiong*), 6g, blast-fried Squama Manitis Pentadactylis (*Shan Jia*), 6g, Herba Ardisiae Japonicae (*Ping Di Mu*), 30g, Herba Lysimachiae Christinae (*Xian Ren Dui Zuo Cao*), 30g, uncooked Fructus Germinatus Hordei Vulgaris (*Mai Ya*), 30g, Lignum Santali Albi (*Tan Xiang*), 1.5g, Rhizoma Corydalis Yanhusuo (*Yan Hu Suo*), 9g, Rhizoma Curcumae Zedoariae (*E Zhu*), 9g, Resina Olibani (*Ru Xiang*), 4.5g

D. Qi vacuity & blood stasis

Main symptoms: A somber yellow complexion, insidious pain in the lateral costal region, upper abdominal distention and fullness which is worse at night, spiritual fatigue, lack of strength, superficial edema of the lower limbs, short, scanty urination, a fat, dark tongue with teeth indentations, and a deep, wiry, forceless pulse

Treatment principles: Boost the qi and transform stasis, move water and open the network vessels

Rx: Radix Astragali Membranacei (*Huang Qi*), 30g, Rhizoma Atractylodis (*Cang Zhu*), 9g, Radix Salviae Miltiorrhizae (*Dan Shen*), 15g, Radix Rubrus Paeoniae Lactiflorae (*Chi Shao*), 9g, Radix Stephaniae Tetrandrae (*Fang Ji*), 9g, Sclerotium Poriae Cocos (*Fu Ling*), 9g, Sclerotium Polypori Umbellati (*Zhu Ling*), 15g, Rhizoma Alismatis (*Ze*

Xie), 9g, Fructus Foeniculi Vulgaris (*Xiao Hui Xiang*), 4.5g, Pericarpium Viridis Citri Reticulatae (*Qing Pi*), 6g, Radix Lateralis Praeparatus Aconiti Carmichaeli (*Fu Zi*), 6g, Cortex Cinnamomi (*Rou Gui*), 1.5g

Secret Essentials

1. In the initial stage, the disease mechanism of hepatitis is chiefly dampness. In the middle stage, it is mainly heat. While in the late stage, it is mainly stasis. However, stasis passes through all these various stages. Therefore, although the treatment principles for treating different types of hepatitis are not the same, it is necessary to take the method of quickening the blood and transforming stasis as the central idea. Thus with half the effort, one may achieve twice the results. For treating dampness, nothing else is better than Rhizoma Atractylodes (*Cang Zhu*). For treating heat, Cornu Rhinocerotis (*Xi Jiao*), Herba Lysimachiae Christinae (*Xian Ren Dui Zuo Cao*), and Herba Ardisiae Japonicae (*Ping Di Mu*) are compatible with the disease mechanism. For transforming stasis, Semen Pruni Persicae (*Tao Ren*), Radix Ligustici Wallichii (*Chuan Xiong*), and Rhizoma Curcumae Zedoariae (*E Zhu*) have particular merit. In terms of the site of the disease, the liver and spleen are important not only in treatment but also in prevention. I commonly use the methods of fortifying the spleen and cultivating earth. This is also effective for preventing the recurrence of the liver diseases. Patients with hepatitis who regularly take the flavor, Rhizoma Atractylodes, can prevent and treat this disease. The rationale is to make replete (*i.e.*, strengthen) the liver by banking earth.

2. In treating liver diseases, it is not appropriate to take too many, too varied, too enriching, or too supplementing medicinals. All these are greatly prohibited during treatment.

13. Chronic Nephritis (*Man Xing Shen Yan*)

In TCM, chronic nephritis is categorized as water swelling (*shui zhong*), low back pain (*yao tong*), and vacuity taxation (*xu lao*). It is believed in TCM that the production of water swelling depends on whether or not the blood flow is uninhibited. For instance, the chapter titled "Piercing to Discipline True & Evil" in the *Ling Shu (Spiritual Pivot)* states:

> When the blood pathways are not free-flowing, one cannot rest in the day. One cannot look up and down easily. Nor can they run about. This disease involves the water.

The *Jin Gui Yao Lue (Essentials from the Golden Cabinet)* states:

> When blood does not flow freely, it will become the water and is called the blood aspect. If channel water is first interrupted and then becomes diseased water, this is called the blood aspect. This disease is difficult to treat. If first water is diseased and then channel water is interrupted, this is called the water aspect. This disease is easy to treat.

All this explains that blood stagnation in the vessels and network vessels may form water swelling. Further, static blood may not only be the cause but also the consequence of water swelling. Physicians in later generations accordingly elaborated on this point. The *Zheng Zhi Hui Bu (Supplement to Patterns & Treatment)* states:

> Stasis swelling skin looks shiny. There appear red traces of blood, showing that blood is transformed into water.

Shen Shi Zhun Sheng Shu (Master Shen's Book on Respecting Life) states:

> Blood is transformed into water. Earth is vanquished and cannot disinhibit water. This leads to stoppage, retention, and non-movement. Retention stagnates in the skin and this produces superficial edema.

The *Xue Zheng Lun (Treatise on Bleeding Patterns)* says: "Patients with blood diseases may also be diseased in water, while those with water diseases may likewise be diseased in blood."

The form in which chronic nephritis begins is not the same. Some patients may not have any marked symptoms at the outset. Only on physical examination is it discovered that there is albuminuria or high blood pressure. After affection with this diseases, most patients manifest symptoms such as fatigue, lack of strength, headache, superficial edema, high blood pressure, and anemia. In a few cases, the arising of this disease is abrupt. Superficial edema is pronounced and there appears large quantities of albumin in the urine. Some patients are asymptomatic until at last there appears the symptoms of uremia, such as vomiting and hemorrhage, and only then do they begin to consult their physician. Chronic nephritis is chiefly manifested by superficial edema, hypertension, abnormal laboratory findings on examination of urine, and damage to kidney function. If superficial edema persists, superficial edema of the eyelids and pitting edema will eventually become pronounced.

Disease causes, disease mechanisms

The occurrence of chronic nephritis is related to the lungs, spleen, and kidneys. Among these, the kidneys are the ruler. The kidneys govern water, treasure the essence, and transform the blood. Blood is capable of nourishing the kidneys. It is also capable of transforming and engendering essence blood. The production of blood cannot be separated from the water fluids. Physiologically, blood and fluids mutually supplement and fill each other. They jointly fulfill the physiological functions of the organism. Pathophysiologically, they also influence each other. Water diseases can extend to the blood, while blood diseases may reach the water. Hence, there is the theory that, "Fluids and blood share a common source." The transportation and movement of the water fluids in the human body depend on the qi transformation of the viscera and bowels. For instance, the lung qi regulates the free-flow. The spleen qi conducts and transports. And the kidney qi steams and soars. Otherwise, the channel qi must necessarily be inhibited, and the channels and vessels must necessarily be static and obstructed. Qi stagnation and blood stasis are thus the root cause of the occurrence of water swelling.

Treatment based on pattern discrimination

A. Stasis & heat struggling & binding

Main symptoms: Water swelling of the cheeks of the face and the four limbs, when pressured, it easily arises, aversion to cold, fever, headache, dizziness, a dry mouth, a bitter taste in the mouth, skin eczema, ceaseless itching, deep yellow urine, amount scanty and hot, a purple red tongue with a yellow, slimy coating, and a wiry, rapid pulse

Treatment principles: Clear heat and resolve toxins, quicken the blood and disinhibit water

Rx: Herba Solani Negri (*Long Gui*), 30g, Herba Duchneseae Indicae (*She Mei*), 30g, Herba Solani Lyrati (*Shu Yang Quan*), 30g, Cortex Phellodendri (*Huang Bai*), 9g, Rhizoma Atractylodis (*Cang Zhu*), 9g, Semen Coicis Lachryma-jobi (*Yi Ren*), 30g, Cortex Radicis Moutan (*Dan Pi*), 9g, uncooked Pollen Typhae (*Pu Huang*), 9g, Radix Salviae Miltiorrhizae (*Dan Shen*), 10 g, Herba Leonuri Heterophylli (*Yi Mu Cao*), 30g, powdered Bombyx Batryticatus (*Jiang Can*), 4.5g, Herba Lycopi Lucidi (*Ze Lan*), 9g, Sclerotium Poriae Cocos (*Fu Ling*), 9g

B. Qi vacuity & blood stasis

Main symptoms: Water swelling in the cheeks, face, and feet which is aggravated by over-taxation, bodily form vacuous and debilitated, fatigue, a sallow yellow complexion, devitalized appetite, epigastric and abdominal distention and falling, low back and knee soreness and pain, inhibited urination and defecation or possible diarrhea, a fat tongue with static patches and a thin, slimy coating, and a wiry, choppy pulse

Treatment principles: Boost the qi and move water, quicken the blood and transform stasis

Rx: Radix Astragali Membranacei (*Huang Qi*), 30g, Radix Codonopsis

Pilosulae (*Dang Shen*), 9g, Rhizoma Atractylodis (*Cang Zhu*), 9g, Rhizoma Atractylodis Macrocephalae (*Bai Zhu*), 9g, Radix Stephaniae Tetrandrae (*Fang Ji*), 9g, Sclerotium Polypori Umbellati (*Zhu Ling*), 9g, Sclerotium Poriae Cocos (*Fu Ling*), 9g, Rhizoma Alismatis (*Ze Xie*), 9g, Ramulus Cinnamomi (*Gui Zhi*), 6g, Pericarpium Citri Reticulatae (*Chen Pi*), 6g, Herba Leonuri Heterophylli (*Yi Mu Cao*), 30g, Radix Ligustici Wallichii (*Chuan Xiong*), 9g, Semen Pruni Persicae (*Tao Ren*), 9g

C. Yang vacuity & blood stasis

Main symptoms: Facial and bodily superfical edema, especially below the waist, pressure causing the skin to be like mud (*i.e.*, pitting edema), a somber, dark complexion, fear of cold, spiritual fatigue, inversion chill of the four limbs, heart palpitations, shortness of breath, bluish purple lips and nails, low back region soreness, heaviness, aching, and pain, inhibited urination, a pale, purple, and fat tongue with a white, slimy coating, and a deep, choppy, forceless pulse

Treatment principles: Warm the kidneys and supplement yang, boost the qi and quicken the blood

Rx: Cornu Cervi (*Lu Jiao Pian*), 9g, Cortex Cinnamomi (*Rou Gui*), 3g, Radix Morindae Officinalis (*Ba Ji Tian*), 9g, Radix Lateralis Praeparatus Aconiti Carmichaeli (*Fu Zi*), 6g, Radix Astragali Membranacei (*Huang Qi*), 12 g, Cortex Eucommiae Ulmoidis (*Du Zhong*), 9g, Sclerotium Polypori Umbellati (*Zhu Ling*), 9g, Sclerotium Poriae Cocos (*Fu Ling*), 9g, Rhizoma Alismatis (*Ze Xie*), 15g, Radix Ligustici Wallichii (*Chuan Xiong*), 6g, Radix Rubrus Paeoniae Lactiflorae (*Chi Shao*), 9g, Semen Pruni Persicae (*Tao Ren*), 9g, Herba Leonuri Heterophylli (*Yi Mu Cao*), 30g

Secret essentials

1. In TCM, chronic nephritis is generally known as water qi disease (*shui qi bing*). This is because damp, turbid substances and blood stasis become mutually bound, obstructing and stagnating the qi mechanism.

Thus qi transformation cannot reach different regions and the kidney loses its sealing and closing function. Since using the methods of quickening the blood and transforming stasis in treating this disease, a break-through has been made in clinical practice.

2. At the beginning of this disease, I like to use Herba Lycopi Lucidi (*Ze Lan*) and Herba Leonuri Heterophylli (*Yi Mu Cao*) to transform blood into water. In the middle stage, I like to use uncooked Pollen Typhae (*Pu Huang*) and Hirudo (*Shui Zhi*) to transform stasis and open the network vessels. These all are efficacious. In the terminal stage, yin congelation is rather severe. Qi and blood circulate irregularly, forming the pattern of block and repulsion. If *Wen Pi Tang* (Warm the Spleen Decoction, *i.e.*, Radix Angelicae Sinensis [*Dang Gui*], 9g, dry Rhizoma Zingiberis [*Gan Jiang*], 2.4g, Radix Lateralis Praeparatus Aconiti Carmichaeli [*Fu Zi*], 9g, Radix Panacis Ginseng [*Ren Shen*], 6g, Radix Glycyrrhizae [*Gan Cao*], 3g, Radix Et Rhizoma Rhei [*Da Huang*], 9g, and Mirabilitum [*Mang Xiao*], 6g) is mixed with Lignum Sappan (*Su Mu*), Flos Carthami Tinctorii (*Hong Hua*), and Semen Pruni Persicae (*Tao Ren*) and is administered to warm yang and transform turbidity, then there is still some hope for treatment. If the stasis heat damages liver/kidney yin, blood heat moves recklessly, while spirit brilliance is depressed. Then the condition will become very critical.

3. In the course of occurrence and development of block and repulsion, spleen/kidney yang vacuity is often taken as the root. In that case, *Fu Gui Ba Bei Wan* (Aconite & Cinnamon Eight Flavors Pills)[10] should be administered, 9g each time, 2 times per day, to stabilize the condition of the disease and prevent its development. This produces a definite effect.

---

[10] These pills are composed of: Radix Lateralis Praeparatus Aconiti Carmichaeli (*Fu Zi*), Ramulus Cinnamomi (*Gui Zhi*), prepared Radix Rehmanniae (*Shu Di*), Radix Dioscoreae Oppositae (*Shan Yao*), Fructus Corni Orricinalis (*Shan Zhu Yu*), Sclerotium Poriae Cocos (*Fu Ling*), Cortex Radicis Moutan (*Dan Pi*), and Rhizoma Alimastis (*Ze Xie*).

14. Uremia (*Niao Du Zheng*)

If the urine is not free-flowing, this is called block. If there is vomiting that does not stop, this is called repulsion. These two may both be observed. Uremia is commonly seen accompanying nephritis. This is mostly due to spleen/kidney dual deficiency. Enduring disease enters the network vessels. Damp heat, stasis, and turbidity join and bind. Qi transformation does not reach the different regions. Thus the patho-condition is very critical. Acute renal function debility and exhaustion may also be caused by drowning or injury from burns.

Disease causes, disease mechanisms

This disease is caused by yang vacuity and yin congelation. Due to stasis turbidity congestion and exuberance, the triple burner qi transformation loses its normalcy. Clear qi is not able to rise and be upborne; while turbid qi cannot obtain precipitation and downbearing. The root is vacuity, while the branch is replete. Thus the pathocondition's nature is complicated and can take many changes.

Treatment based on pattern discrimination

A. Spleen/kidney yang vacuity

Main symptoms: A bright white or dark and stagnant complexion, lack of warmth in the four limbs, low back and knee soreness and weakness, legs and feet aching and painful, superficial edema marked below the waist, nausea, vomiting, no thought for food, and scanty urination or even anuria; however urination may be clear, long, and frothy. The pulse is deep and fine. The tongue coating is thin and like white jade.

Treatment principles: Warm the spleen and boost the kidneys, quicken the blood and transform stasis

Rx: Bland Radix Lateralis Praeparatus Aconiti Carmichaeli (*Dan Fu Pian*), 9g, Ramulus Cinnamomi (*Gui Zhi*), 4.5g, Rhizoma Atractylodis

(*Cang Zhu*), 9g, Rhizoma Atractylodis Macrocephalae (*Bai Zhu*), 9g, Rhizoma Alismatis (*Ze Xie*), 9g, Sclerotium Polypori Umbellati (*Zhu Ling*), 9g, Sclerotium Poriae Cocos (*Fu Ling*), 9g, Radix Ligustici Wallichii (*Chuan Xiong*), 9g, Flos Carthami Tinctorii (*Hong Hua*), 9g, Rhizoma Pinelliae Ternatae (*Ban Xia*), 9g, Pericarpium Citri Reticulatae (*Chen Pi*), 6g, Herba Leonuri Heterophylli (*Yi Mu Cao*), 30g, Fructus Foeniculi Vulgaris (*Xiao Hui Xiang*), 2.4g, Semen Trigonellae Foenigraeci (*Hu Lu Ba*), 9g, Folium Eupatorii Chinensis (*Liu Yue Xue*), 30g, Semen Glycinis Hispidae (*Hei Da Dou*), 30g

B. Turbidity flooding the triple burner

Main symptoms: A lusterless complexion, nausea, vomiting, lack of appetite, abdominal distention, a slimy mouth and sweet taste, stools not free-flowing, heaviness of the four limbs, a fat, pale tongue body with teeth indentations on its edges, and a deep, fine pulse

Treatment principles: Warm yang and assist transportation, transform stasis and discharge turbidity

Rx: Uncooked Rhizoma Pinelliae Ternatae (*Ban Xia*), 30g, decoct in advance 2 hours, Flos Inulae (*Xuan Fu Hua*), 9g, wrapped during decoction, Haematitum (*Dai Zhe Shi*), 30g, uncooked Rhizoma Zingiberis (*Sheng Jiang*), 5 slices, ginger(-processed) Sichuan Rhizoma Coptidis Chinensis (*Chuan Lian*), 3g, Fructus Evodiae Rutecarpae (*Dan Wu Zhu*), 2.4g, Sclerotium Poriae Cocos (*Fu Ling*), 9g, Cortex Magnoliae Officinalis (*Chuan Po*), 6g, Folium Eupatorii Chinensis (*Liu Yue Xue*), 30g, Semen Glycinis Hispidae (*Hei Da Dou*), 30g

C. Liver wind internally stirring

Main symptoms: Urinary blockage, trembling fingers, headache, gum redness and swelling, oral ulcers, skin itching, in severe cases, spirit darkness (*i.e.*, syncope), tremors, and agitation, worry, and restlessness, a dry, scarlet tongue with a scorched yellow coating, a curled upward or trembling tongue, and a fine, weak, rapid pulse

Treatment principles: Suppress yang and search wind, quicken the blood and transform stasis

Rx: *Zi Xian Chi* (紫见齿), 30g, mix-fried Carapax Amydae Sinensis (*Bie Jia*), 15g, Plastrum Testudinis (*Gui Ban*), 15g, fresh Herba Dendrobii (*Shi Hu*), 9g, Ramulus Uncariae Cum Uncis (*Shuang Gou*), 15g, Radix Scrophulariae Ningpoensis (*Xuan Shen*), 15g, Radix Et Rhizoma Rhei (*Da Huang*), 9g, Sclerotium Pararadicis Poriae Cocos (*Fu Ling Shen*), 9g, Tuber Ophiopogonis Japonicae (*Mai Dong*), 9g, Semen Plantaginis (*Che Qian Zi*), 9g, Radix Achyranthis Bidentatae (*Niu Xi*), 9g, uncooked Radix Rehmanniae (*Sheng Di*), 15g

Secret Essentials

1. For uremia, I commonly use the therapy of discharging turbidity from the intestinal tract. In order to do this, decoct Folium Eupatorii Chinensis (*Liu Yue Xue*), 30g, and uncooked Radix Et Rhizoma Rhei (*Da Huang*), 30g, down to 150ml of liquid. Use this as a retention enema, 1 time per day. This produces a good effect in reducing retention of ureic nitrogen and creatinine.

2. During the relaxing and resolving period of uremia (*i.e.*, during remission), decoct Rhizoma Atractylodis Macrocephalae (*Bai Zhu*), 60g, with rice soup and take 1 time per day. This treatment can lengthen the period of remission.

15. Chronic Pulmonary Heart Disease (*Man Xing Fei Quan Xing Xin Zang Bing*)

In TCM, pulmonary heart disease is categorized as lung distention (*fei zhang*). The term lung distention is first seen in the *Nei Jing (Inner Classic), Ling Shu (Spiritual Pivot)*, "Treatise on Distention" which says, "Lung distention means vacuity, fullness, panting, and cough." The *Jin Gui Yao Lue (Essential Prescriptions from the Golden Chamber)* further points out in regards to the main symptoms of this disease that:

Cough and ascending qi produce lung distention. The person pants and their eyes look as if they had fallen out.

Physicians in different dynasties have written numerous dissertations on the pathophysiology of this disease. Among these, the theory of Zhu Dan-xi is, in particular, full of original ideas. He said:

> With lung distention there is cough, turning to the left or to the right, and inability to sleep. Phlegm is mixed with static blood and hinders the qi. Thus this disease. It is appropriate to nourish the blood so as to course, stir, and level the qi and to downbear fire and course the liver so as to clear phlegm.

He advanced the view that the pathophysiology of this disease is phlegm stasis obstructing and hindering the lung qi. He first recommended the using *Si Ni Tang* (Four Counterflows Decoction) plus Semen Pruni Persciae (*Tao Ren*) for treatment, thus setting a precedent for applying the therapy of quickening the blood and transforming stasis to treat lung distention. Recently, with the deepening of research on the pattern of static blood and on the methods of quickening the blood and transforming stasis, we have further knowledge of the role that static blood plays in the pathophysiology of this disease. In 1977, the Second National Conference for the Speciality in Pulmonary Heart Diseases revised the *Man Xing Quan Xing Xin Zang Bing Zhong Xi Yi Jie He Biang Zheng Fen Xing He Zhi Liao Quan Ze (Principles of Integrated Chinese-Western Medical Pattern Discrimination & Treatment of Chronic Heart Diseases)*, pointing out that:

> Pulmonary heart disease may be divided into the stage of remission and that of acute attack. Qi vacuity and blood stasis may pass through these two stages from the beginning to the end. The treatment methods of quickening the blood and transforming stasis may be appropriately applied during both of these stages.

Disease causes, disease mechanisms

Pulmonary heart disease is located in the two viscera of the lungs and heart. However, it extends to the spleen and kidneys. The heart and lungs are both in the upper burner. The heart is "the sovereign ruler." It governs the constructive and blood. The lungs are "the prime minister" and govern the defensive qi. The lungs help the heart to move the blood vessels, while the heart depends on the lung qi to transport and spread through the whole body. Therefore, if the lungs and heart are diseased, confusion and chaos of the qi and blood must necessarily appear, leading to the production of static blood. Thus, the pathophysiology of static blood in pulmonary heart disease may be summed up in three conditions: First, if cough and panting endure for days, lung qi will become deficient and suffer detriment. This makes difficult its passing through and free flow within the heart vessels. Because blood does not move uninhibitedly, stasis occurs. Secondly, if disease lingers on, it first is in the channels but later enters the network vessels, forming stasis. And third, pulmonary heart disease is mostly seen in the elderly. At 60, heart qi becomes debilitated. At 80, lung qi becomes debilitated. Thus, as the age rises in a person, qi becomes debilitated, leading to lack of force in the transportation of blood. The movement of blood loses its normalcy and the vessels and pathways are obstructed by stasis. After some time, when the function of the heart and lungs lose their capacity for compensation, the physical signs of respiratory failure and heart failure will appear. The complexion looks ashen and dark. The breath is short and the patient cannot lie down. There is superficial edema of the lower limbs. If severe, there is superficial edema of the entire body. The lips and nails are purple. The tongue is purple and the pulse is choppy. These are all obvious symptoms of the pattern of static blood.

Treatment based on pattern discrimination

A. Phlegm stasis congesting the lungs

Main symptoms: Cough, qi panting, excessive phlegm like white froth, movement results in panting and wheezing, chest oppression, lung distention, a purple tongue, especially on the two edges, distended and engorged veins beneath the tongue, a thin, white tongue coating, and a wiry, slippery pulse

Treatment principles: Transform phlegm and level panting, quicken the blood and transform stasis

Rx: Radix Angelicae Sinensis (*Dang Gui*), 9g, Flos Carthami Tinctorii (*Hong Hua*), 9g, Radix Bupleuri (*Chai Hu*), 6g, Radix Platycodi Grandiflori (*Jie Geng*), 6g, Radix Ligustici Wallichii (*Chuan Xiong*), 6g, Radix Achyranthis Bidentatae (*Niu Xi*), 6g, Radix Salviae Miltiorrhizae (*Dan Shen*), 15g, Cortex Radicis Mori Albi (*Sang Pi*), 9g, Semen Pruni Armeniacae (*Xing Ren*), 9g, lime(-processed) Rhizoma Pinelliae Ternatae (*Fa Ban Xia*), 9g, Radix Glycyrrhizae (*Gan Cao*), 3g, Fructus Citri Seu Ponciri (*Zhi Qiao*), 6g, Semen Lepidii (*Ting Li Zi*), 9g

B. Phlegm heat mixed with stasis

Main symptoms: Cough, panting, chest fullness, forceful breathing, yellow or white phlegm which is pasty and sticky and difficult to spit up, vexation and agitation, oral thirst, yellowish red urination, dry, bound stools, a purple red tongue with a yellow, slimy coating, and a slippery, rapid pulse

Treatment principles: Clear the lungs and break up phlegm, quicken the blood and transform stasis

Rx: Flos Inulae (*Xuan Fu Hua*), 9g, Rhizoma Phragmitis Communis (*Lu Gen*), 30g, Folium Eriobotryae Japonicae (*Bi Ba Ye*), 9g, Herba Houttuyniae Cordatae (*Yu Xing Cao*), 30g, Fructus Trichosanthis Kirlowii (*Quan Gua Lou*), 18g, Radix Scutellariae Baicalensis (*Huang Qin*), 9g, lime(-processed) Rhizoma Pinelliae Ternatae (*Fa Ban Xia*), 9g, Radix Rubrus Paeoniae Lactiflorae (*Chi Shao*), 9g, Cortex Radicis Moutan (*Dan Pi*), 9g, Semen Lepidii (*Ting Li Zi*), 9g, green Bulbus Allii Fistulosi (*Cong Bai*), 3 stalks

C. Phlegm stasis confounding the heart

Main symptoms: Dull expression, abstracted spirit orientation or vexation and agitation and uneasiness, random motion of the hands and feet, tremors, possible drowsiness and stupor, shortness of breath, a phlegmy sound when breathing, purple lips, a dark red or pale purple tongue with either a white, slimy or yellow, slimy coating, and a wiry, rapid, bound pulse

Treatment principles: Transform phlegm and open the portals, quicken the blood and open the network vessels

Rx: Lime(-processed) Rhizoma Pinelliae Ternatae (*Fa Ban Xia*), 9g, Rhizoma Coptidis Chinensis (*Chuan Lian*), 3g, Pericarpium Citri Reticulatae (*Chen Pi*), 6g, Sclerotium Poriae Cocos (*Fu Ling*), 9g, bile(-processed) Rhizoma Arisaematis (*Dan Xing*), 6g, Fructus Immaturus Citri Seu Ponciri (*Zhi Shi*), 9g, Rhizoma Acori Graminei (*Chang Pu*), 9g, Radix Polygalae Tenuifoliae (*Yuan Zhi*), 9g, Caulis in Taeniis Bambusae (*Zhu Ru*), 6g, Tuber Curcumae (*Yu Jin*), 9g, Radix Salviae Miltiorrhizae (*Dan Shen*), 15g, Radix Rubrus Paeoniae Lactiflorae (*Chi Shao*), 9g, Radix Glycyrrhizae (*Gan Cao*), 3g, *Su He Xiang Wan* (Styrax Pills), 1/2 bolus, *Hou Zao San* (Monkey Pad Powder), 0.6g (These two flavors, *i.e.*, medicines, should be mixed together and washed down with the decoction.)

D. Yang vacuity & blood stasis

Main symptoms: A somber, dark complexion, fear of cold, liking for warmth, cough, qi panting, excessive white, frothy phlegm, a hoarse voice, and qi fright. In severe cases, the mouth is opened wide to breath and the shoulders are raised. There is superficial edema of the limbs and body. The tongue is dark purple, and the pulse is vacuous and fine.

Treatment principles: Warm yang and boost the qi, quicken the blood and transform stasis

Rx: Radix Codonopsis Pilosulae (*Dang Shen*), 15g, Radix Astragali Membranacei (*Huang Qi*), 15g, Lignum Aquilariae Agallochae (*Chen Xiang*), 0.9g, prepared Radix Rehmanniae (*Shu Di*), 15g, Fructus Schizandrae Chinensis (*Wu Wei Zi*), 6g, Radix Angelicae Sinensis (*Dang Gui*), 9g, Radix Ligustici Wallichii (*Chuan Xiong*), 6g, Flos Carthami Tinctorii (*Hong Hua*), 9g, Radix Salviae Miltiorrhizae (*Dan Shen*), 15g, Rhizoma Atractylodis Macrocephalae (*Bai Zhu*), 10 g, Rhizoma Pinelliae Ternatae (*Ban Xia*), 9g, Radix Lateralis Praeparatus Aconiti Carmichaeli (*Fu Zi*), 9g, *Kan Ya* (坎爭), 2 stalks

Secret Essentials

In this disease, the root is vacuous, while the branch is replete. Phlegm stasis obstructs the qi mechanism, and depuration and downbearing lose their command. Vacuity cannot be supplemented, while repletion cannot bear attacking. This is like a thorn in the hand. Because stasis passes through the whole course of this disease, therefore, in treating it, one should correspondingly attach importance to quickening the blood and transforming stasis. I use commonly use Hirudo (*Shui Zhi*), typically at 3g per decoction. This is powdered and divided into two 1.5g doses which are swallowed down with the decoction. This is able to improve symptoms due to lack of oxygen. However, because Hirudo's nature is cold, it should be swallowed along with an equal amount of powdered Lignum Dalbergiae Odoriferae (*Jiang Xiang*) or powdered Lignum Aquilariae Agallochae (*Chen Xiang*) which should be evenly mixed up with the pulverized Hirudo. Those with chronic pulmonary heart disease may take powdered Hirudo and powdered Radix Panacis Ginseng (*Ren Shen*) administered together. These medicinals can prevent diseases of the lungs, heart, and brain.

16. Prostatic Hyperplasia (*Qian Lie Xian Zeng Sheng Zheng*)

Prostatic hyperplasia is also known as prostatic hypertrophy. It is a common male geriatric disease, and occurs most frequently in the people over 50 years of age, with its incidence peaking between 60-70 years of age.

Prostatic hyperplasia is categorized as dribbling urinary block (*long bi*) in TCM. In the *Nei Jing (Inner Classic)*, there are already records of a similar condition. The chapter titled "Diffusing & Brigthening the Five Qi" in the *Su Wen (Simple Questions)* states:

> When the bladder is inhibited, it is *long*. When it does not restrain (the urine), it is involuntary discharge.

"The Treatise on Root & Branch in Disease" in the *Su Wen (Simple Questions)* further says, "When bladder is diseased, urination is closed." The *Yi Xue Gang Mu (Detailed Outline of the Study of Medicine)* from the Ming Dynasty gives a detailed account of this disease. It states:

> When *long* and *bi* are mentioned together, they mean just one disease. If they are discussed separately, then there is the difference between sudden attack and persistent affection, for *bi* or blockage means sudden attack of the disease. It is called retention of urine which cannot dribble or drip out. It is popularly known as lack of free flow of urination. *Long* indicates an enduring disease. Each day, urine dribbles out several tens of times or even one hundred times.

Not a few physicians in different dynasties have thought that static blood is a very important cause for the occurrence of this disease. For instance, Zhang Zhong-jing in the Han Dynasty invented *Pu Tan San* (Dandelion Ash Powder) and *Hua Shi Bai Yu San* (Talcum White Fish Powder). These are quickening the blood and transforming stasis medicinals taken internally for the treatment inhibited urination. In the Ming Dynasty, Zhang Jing-yue said, "Either due to vanquished essence or acccumulation of blood, the water pathways are obstructed and blocked and are thus not free-flowing." According to records, Fructus Gleditschiae Chinensis (*Zao Jiao*), Bulbus Allii Fistulosi (*Cong Tou*), and Semen Vaccariae Segetalis (*Wang Bu Liu Xing*) can be decocted together in.a tub. The patient is asked to soak so as to steam and wash the lower abdomen and lower body. If this sitz bath lasts long and hot

steam reaches the interior, then congestion and blockage will spontaneously be opened. This means that moving stasis and scattering nodulations with medicinals that quicken the blood can open strangury (*i.e.*,
dribbling) and open *bi* (*i.e.*, blockage).

Disease causes, disease mechanisms

In the pattern of dribbling urinary block, although the site of the disease
is in the bladder, in fact, this disease is closely related to the kidney qi.
The kidneys govern water fluids and are in charge of urination and
defecation. The bladder rules the storage of urine. If kidney viscus qi
transformation loses its normalcy, then opening and closing will be
beyond limit, and the bladder will be inhibited. Consequently, *long*
(dribbling) or *bi* (blockage) will occur during urination. Clinically, it
has been discovered that pathological changes in other viscera and
bowels may also lead to the occurrence of this disease. For instance, if
lung qi loses its downbearing, fluid and humor transportation and
spreading loses its regulation and reaching. If spleen qi does not upbear,
damp heat congests and gathers in the lower burner. If the liver loses its
coursing and discharge, qi and blood stasis will obstruct the urinary
tract and genitals. Although the causes of this disease are numerous, the
disease mechanism is nothing other than qi and blood congestion and
stagnation.

In the elderly, kidney yang is insufficient and life gate fire is debilitated.
Thus it is said, "Without yang, yin cannot be engendered." Hence the
bladder qi transformation has no authority. It is possible for heat to
accumulate in the lower burner. If this endures for many days and is not
cured, fluids and humors are consumed and suffer detriment and kidney
yin becomes insufficient. This then leads to what is meant by, "Without
yin, yang cannot be transformed." All this may give rise to dribbling
urinary block. The disease mechanism also lies in inhibition of the qi
mechanism, and static blood obstructing internally.

In the initial stage of this disease, the symptoms of polyuria or nocturnia occur. However, with aggravation of prostatic hyperplasia, difficult urination becomes the most prominent symptom. Those with difficult urination must wait rather long before they can pass urine which is discharged slowly, shoots only a short distance, and even dribbles. Because it cannot be completely discharged, residual urine gradually accumulates, thus gradually aggravating polyuria. Conversely, even incontinence may occur. In medicine, this is known as complete suppression of urination or overflowing incontinence. If these symptoms persist and cannot be improved, they will lead to detriment of kidney function and cause uremia.

Treatment based on pattern discrimination

A. Qi stagnation & blood stasis

Main symptoms: Dribbling and dripping of urination, terminal dribbling, astringency and pain in the penis, pain radiating to the lower abdomen, essence spirit worry and depression, possible heart vexation or tendency to anger, a purple red tongue with a thin, yellow coating, and a wiry, choppy pulse

Treatment principles: Disinhibit urination and open blockage, quicken the blood and transform stasis

Rx: Lignum Aquilariae Agallochae (*Chen Xiang*), 3g, Pericarpium Citri Reticulatae (*Chen Pi*), 6g, rootlets of Radix Angelicae Sinensis (*Gui Wei*), 9g, Radix Achyranthis Bidentatae (*Niu Xi*), 9g, Semen Vaccariae Segetalis (*Wang Bu Liu Xing*), 9g, Folium Pyrrosiae (*Shi Wei*), 15g, Semen Abutilonis Seu Malvae (*Dong Gui Zi*), 9g, Talcum (*Hua Shi*), 9g, Cortex Radicis Moutan (*Dan Pi*), 9g, Fructus Gardeniae Jasminoidis (*Shan Zhi*), 9g, Semen Pistachionis (*Kai Xin Guo*), 9g, Semen Pruni Persicae (*Tao Ren*), 9g

B. Stasis obstructing the bladder

Main symptoms: Urinating drop by drop, fine, thready urination, in severe cases, obstruction, blockage, and no free flow, aching and pain in the lower abdomen and perineum, pain radiating to the testicles, a purple, dark tongue or possible static patches, and fine, wiry pulse

Treatment principles: Dispel stasis and scatter nodulation, clear and disinhibit the water pathways

Rx: Rhizoma Cimicifugae (*Sheng Ma*), 9g, Radix Angelicae Sinensis (*Dang Gui*), 9g, blast-fried Squama Manitis Pentadactylis (*Shan Jia*), 6g, Semen Pruni Persicae (*Tao Ren*), 9g, wine-processed Radix Et Rhizoma Rhei (*Jun*), 9g, Mirabilitum (*Mang Xiao*), 3g, uncooked Radix Rehmanniae (*Sheng Di*), 12g, Cortex Cinnamomi (*Rou Gui*), 1.5g, Flos Carthami Tinctorii (*Hong Hua*), 9g, Radix Achyranthis Bidentatae (*Niu Xi*), 9g, Rhizoma Curcumae Zedoariae (*E Zhu*), 9g, Secretio Moschi Moschiferi (*She Xiang*), 0.1g, swallowed down with the decoction

C. Damp heat & stasis binding

Main symptoms: Numerous, frequent, short, and astringent urination, urinary urgency, urinary pain, constant feeling of the need to urinate, turbid, cloudy urine, lower abdominal and perineal distention and pain, dry, bound stools, a purple tongue with a yellow coating, and a wiry, rapid pulse

Treatment principles: Clear heat and disinhibit dampness, quicken the blood and open the network vessels

Rx: Caulis Akebiae Mutong (*Mu Tong*), 4.5g, Semen Plantaginis (*Che Qian Zi*), 9g, Rhizoma Dioscoreae Hypoglaucae (*Bi Xie*), 9g, Herba Dianthi (*Qu Mai*), 9g, Fructus Gardeniae Jasminoidis (*Shan Zhi*), 9g, Talcum (*Hua Shi*), 9g, Radix Et Rhizoma Rhei (*Da Huang*), 6g, rootlets of Radix Glycyrrhizae (*Gan Cao Xiao*), 3g, Semen Vaccariae Segetalis (*Wang Bu Liu Xing*), 9g, Rhizoma Polygoni Cuspidati (*Hu Zhang*), 9g,

Radix Salviae Miltiorrhizae (*Dan Shen*), 15g, Rhizoma Anemarrhenae 9g, Cortex Phellodendri (*Huang Bai*), 9g, Rhizoma Cimicifugae (*Sheng Ma*), 9g, Semen Pruni Persicae (*Tao Ren*), 9g

D. Yang vacuity & blood stasis

Main symptoms: Lack of force in expelling urine, dribbling and dripping or uneasy urination, low back and knee chilly pain, atony, weakness, aching, and flaccidity, spirit color timid (*i.e.*, facial color pale), heel pain, a purple tongue with a white coating, and a deep, fine, choppy pulse

Treatment principles: Warm and open kidney yang, quicken the blood and transform stasis

Rx: Radix Lateralis Praeparatus Aconiti Carmichaeli (*Dan Fu Pian*), 9g, Cortex Cinnamomi (*Rou Gui*), 1.5g, prepared Radix Rehmanniae (*Shu Di*), 15g, Semen Trigonellae Foeni-graeci (*Hu Lu Ba*), 9g, Semen Pruni Persicae (*Tao Ren*), 9g, Radix Achyranthis Bidentatae (*Niu Xi*), 9g, Cortex Radicis Moutan (*Dan Pi*), 9g, Radix Rubrus Paeoniae Lactiflorae (*Chi Shao*), 9g, Radix Salviae Miltiorrhizae (*Dan Shen*), 15g, Sclerotium Poriae Cocos (*Fu Ling*), 9g, Semen Vaccariae Segetalis (*Wang Bu Liu Xing*), 9g, Rhizoma Cimicifugae (*Sheng Ma*), 6g, Radix Angelicae Sinensis (*Dang Gui*), 9g

Secret Essentials

1. In treating this disease, one should grasp its two important key points: 1) the qi transformation function and 2) quickening the blood and transforming stasis. Qi transformation requires not only disinhibition and downbearing of qi but also that one make good use of supplementing and upbearing qi. The central qi in the elderly often falls downward or there is a tendency for qi to gather in the lower warmer. Therefore, I often add the medicinal Rhizoma Cimicifugae (*Sheng Ma*) to the formula. When one lifts the pot and uncovers the lid, one can get as prompt an effect as observing the shadow as soon as the pole is lifted.

For quickening the blood and transforming stasis as well as softening the hard, one should use Semen Vaccariae Segetalis (*Wang Bu Liu Xing*), blast-fried Squama Manitis Pentadactylis (*Shan Jia*), and Rhizoma Curcumae Zedoariae (*E Zhu*) which are simultaneously mild and drastic medicinals of wonderful effect.

2. This disease often relapses. During the period of remission, one should regularly take *Jin Gui Shen Qi Wan* (Golden Chamber Kidney Qi Pills) and *Bu Zhong Yi Qi Wan* (Supplementing the Middle & Boosting the Qi Pills). These two kinds of pills are alternately administered, 9g each time, 2 times per day. These medicines help to increase the qi transformation function and lengthen the period of remission. However, during the period of acute attack, it is necessary to carry out treatment according to pattern discrimination.

3. If the disease is complicated by lung heat, I like to use *Ma Xing Shi Gan Tang* (Ephedra, Armeniaca, Gypsum, & Licorice Decoction): Herba Ephedrae (*Ma Huang*), 6g, Semen Pruni Armeniacae (*Xing Ren*), 9g, Gypsum Fibrosum (*Shi Gao*), 30g, uncooked Radix Glycyrrhizae (*Gan Cao*), 3g. The lungs are the upper source of water. When the source is cleared, the flow will naturally be long.

4. *Zi Shen Tong Guan Wan* (Enrich the Kidneys & Open the Barrier Pills)[11] are also effective for this disease, 9g each time, 2 times per day.

17. Psychological Disease (*Jing Shen Bing*)

Psychological disease refers to trouble in the cerebral mental activities caused by harmful factors inside and outside the body. Its clinical manifestations are abnormal mental activities in cognition, sentiment, will, and behavior. It belongs to the category of mania and withdrawl

---

[11] These are comprised of: Cortex Phellodendri (*Huang Bai*), 30g, Rhizoma Anemarrhenae (*Zhi Mu*), 30g, and Cortex Cinnamomi (*Rou Gui*), 4.5 g. These are ground into ppowder and made into pills with honey.

(*dian kuang*) in TCM. The ancients already knew that its occurrence is related to static blood. The *Nei Jing (Inner Classic)* says, "Blood is the spirit qi" and "The vessels contain the spirit." This explains from the physiological point of view, the relationship between blood and the spirit. It further states:

> When blood is mixed with yin, while qi is mingled with yang, then fright and mania will occur...

and,

> If blood has a surplus, anger will occur. If it is insufficient, this leads to fear.

From the point of view of pathophysiology, this suggests that imbalance in qi and blood, yin and yang can lead to essence spirit (*i.e.*, psychological) and emotional orientation diseases. In the *Shang Han Lun (Treatise on Damage Due to Cold)*, there are passages where "heat binding in the bladder", "heat entering the blood chamber", and "retained of blood" are all clearly spoken of in terms of the relationship between mania and blood disease. For instance:

> If *tai yang* disease is not resolved, heat will bind in the bladder and the person seems mad. Blood will spontaneously be precipitated... If there is lower abdominal tension and binding, it is all right to attack and precipitate, (in which case,) *Tao He Cheng Qi Tang* (Persica Order the Qi Decoction) is appropriate...

> In *tai yang* disease, the body is yellow, the pulse is deep and bound, the lower abdomen is hard, and urination is inhibited. This is due to static blood. If the urination is spontaneously disinhibited while the patient looks mad, this means that a blood pattern is occuring. *Di Dang Tang* (Resistance Decoction) rules this.

Wang Qing-ren in the Qing Dynasty advanced the view that blood stasis renders it impossible for the cerebral qi to connect with viscera and bowel qi, thus causing mania and withdrawal. This has enabled a breakthrough in the treatment of psychological diseases in recent years.

Disease causes, disease mechanisms

The disease causes of essence spirit disease are chiefly damage by the seven emotions, such as anger, fright, fear or excessive sadness or joy, worry and desires which are unfulfilled, and natural endowment of eccentrically yin or yang temperament. All these may elicit the occurrence of psychological disease whenever one is frightened or mentally/emotionally stimulated. The influence of damage by the seven emotions on the qi is marked. "The Treatise on Pain" in the *Su Wen (Simple Questions)* states:

> Anger and qi goes upward. Joy and qi is relaxed (*i.e.*, to the point of being slack or retarded). Grief and the qi is dispersed. Fear and the qi goes downward. Cold and the qi is restrained. Heat and qi is discharged. Fright and qi is chaotic. Taxation and qi is consumed. Thinking (as in worry) and the qi is bound.

In sum, excesses of the seven emotions can lead to confusion and chaos in organic functions and loss of normalcy in the essence spirit. Qi and blood are mutually bound and mutually tied together. Whether qi or blood is diseased, that will automatically influence the other side. Therefore, if the seven emotions cause damage, qi depression enduring for many days will necessarily cause blood stasis. Qi and blood congelation and stagnation and loss of regularity of the visceral qi and yin and yang is, therefore, the main disease mechanism of this disease.

Treatment based on pattern discrimination

A. Liver fire mixed with stasis

Main symptoms: Mania, agitation, restlessness, incessant crying and scolding, destroying things and beating others, impetuosity, easy anger, a red face and eyes, scaly skin, lower abdominal binding and tension, hardness, fullness, aching and pain which refuses pressure, constipation, a purple tongue with a dry, yellow coating, and a deep, replete or wiry, choppy pulse

Treatment principles: Open the bowels and drain fire, quicken the blood and dispel stasis

Rx: Semen Pruni Persicae (*Tao Ren*), 12g, Radix Et Rhizoma Rhei (*Da Huang*), 9g, Mirabilitum (*Mang Xiao*), 6g, dissovled after the other medicinals are decocted, Radix Angelicae Sinensis (*Dang Gui*), 9g, Radix Gentianae Scabrae (*Long Dan Cao*), 9g, Fructus Gardeniae Jasminoidis (*Shan Zhi*), 9g, Rhizoma Coptidis Chinensis (*Huang Lian*), 4.5g, Radix Scutellariae Baicalensis (*Huang Qin*), 9g, Cortex Phellodendri (*Huang Bai*), 9g, Radix Saussureae Seu Vladimiriae (*Mu Xiang*), 4.5g, Radix Glycyrrhizae (*Gan Cao*), 3g

B. Qi stagnation & blood stasis

Main symptoms: Essence spirit depression, sulleness, easy suspicion, heart vexation, loss of sleep, chaotic dreams, an obstructed sensation in the throat, bluish purple lips, a purple tongue, and a wiry, choppy pulse

Treatment principles: Rectify the qi and resolve depression, quicken the blood and transform stasis

Rx: Radix Bupleuri (*Chai Hu*), 6g, Radix Angelicae Sinensis (*Dang Gui*), 9g, Radix Rubrus Paeoniae Lactiflorae (*Chi Shao*), 9g, Flos Carthami Tinctorii (*Hong Hua*), 9g, Semen Pruni Persicae (*Tao Ren*), 9g, uncooked Radix Rehmanniae (*Sheng Di*), 9g, Fructus Citri Seu Ponciri (*Zhi Qiao*), 6g, Radix Platycodi Grandiflori (*Jie Geng*), 4.5g, Radix Achyranthis Bidentatae (*Niu Xi*), 6g, Rhizoma Acori Graminei (*Chang Pu*), 9g, Rhizoma Pinelliae Ternatae (*Ban Xia*), 9g, Radix Glycyrrhizae (*Gan Cao*), 3g

C. Phlegm & stasis joining & binding

Main symptoms: Mental dullness, a bland, expressionless affect, disordered speech or mumbling soliloquy, instability of joy and anger, sudden falling and fainting, phlegmy sounds in the throat, vomiting white froth, chest and diaphragamtic oppression, no thought for food and drink, a purple tongue with a slimy coating, and a wiry, slippery pulse

Treatment principles: Quicken the blood and resolve depression, transform phlegm and open the portals

Rx: Semen Pruni Persicae (*Tao Ren*), 9g, Flos Carthami Tinctorii (*Hong Hua*), 9g, Radix Rubrus Paeoniae Lactiflorae (*Chi Shao*), 9g, Radix Ligustici Wallichii (*Chuan Xiong*), 9g, Fructus Citri Seu Ponciri (*Zhi Qiao*), 6g, lime(-processed) Rhizoma Pinelliae Ternatae (*Fa Ban Xia*), 9g, Pericarpium Citri Reticulatae (*Chen Pi*), 6g, Sclerotium Poriae Cocos (*Fu Ling*), 9g, Caulis in Taeniis Bambusae (*Zhu Ru*), 6g, Radix Glycyrrhizae (*Gan Cao*), 3g, Rhizoma Acori Graminei (*Chang Pu*), 9g, Tuber Curcumae (*Yu Jin*), 9g, Radix Polygalae Tenuifoliae (*Yuan Zhi*), 9g, Radix Salviae Miltiorrhizae (*Dan Shen*), 15g, powdered Succinum (*Hu Po*), 0.6g, washed down by the other decocted medicinals

D. Qi vacuity & blood stasis

Main symptoms: Essence spirit abstraction, lack of self-control, heart palpitations, easily frightened, sadness and willingness to weep, fatigue, lack of spirit, no thought for food and drink, a pale purplish tongue with a white coating, and a fine, choppy pulse

Treatment principles: Boost the qi and stabilize the spirit, quicken the blood and nourish the heart

Rx: Fructus Levis Tritici Aestivi (*Huai Xiao Mai*), 30g, Fructus Zizyphi Jujubae (*Da Zao*), 5 pieces, Radix Glycyrrhizae (*Gan Cao*), 4.5g, Bulbus Lilii (*Bai He*), 9g, Tuber Ophiopogonis Japonicae (*Mai Dong*), 9g, Radix Salviae Miltiorrhizae (*Dan Shen*), 15g, Radix Polygalae Tenuifoliae (*Yuan Zhi*), 6g, Semen Biotae Orientalis (*Bai Zi Ren*), 9g, Semen Zizyphi Spinosae (*Zao Ren*), 9g, Radix Rubrus Paeoniae Lactiflorae (*Chi Shao*), 12g, Radix Ligustici Wallichii (*Chuan Xiong*), 9g, Radix Angelicae Sinensis (*Dang Gui*), 9g, Magnetitum (*Ci Shi*), 30g, Dens Draconis (*Long Chi*), 30g

Secret Essentials

1. During an uncontrollable attack of mania and agitation, it is all right to use large doses of Rhizoma Coptidis Chinensis (*Huang Lian*). Each formula may contain 9g of this medicinal. *Dian Zheng Long Hu Dan* (Mania Condition Dragon Tiger Elixir) prepared by the Shanghai drugstore Cai Tong De is also quite effective. Take 1 bolus each time, 1 time per day.

2. In treating essence spirit loss of normalcy (*i.e.*, mental/emotional disorders), one should take as the basis medicinals for quickening the blood and transforming stasis. Then, according to pattern discrimination, add and subtract medicinals. Because the heart governs the spirit brilliance, therefore, in treating spirit brilliance bewilderment and chaos, the blood is the ruler. In treating this disease, one can regularly use *Xue Fu Zhu Yu Tang* (Blood Mansion Dispel Stasis Decoction) plus Rhizoma Acori Graminei (*Chang Pu*), 9g. There are quite a few effective cases for reference. Each week the patient should take 2 packets. This is effective for preventing the recurrence of this disease.

18. Senile Dementia (*Lao Nian Qi Chi Dai*)

Senile dementia is also known as senile psychosis. This refers to essence spirit disease which occurs before or after 65 years of age. Its pathological change is extensive cerebral atrophy which is marked in the frontal lobe. The weight of the brain is at least 100g lighter than that of a normal elderly person. The neurons are atrophic, and the number and quality of nerve cells are reduced. Because the average length of human life has been prolonged, the incidence of senile dementia is gradually rising. According to the viewpoint that "Purity means intelligence, while miscellany means interruption", through years of exploration, I have come to believe that the root of this disease is static blood obstructing the mansion of the clear spirit. Therefore, using the methods of quickening the blood and transforming stasis, I have gotten satisfactory therapeutic results, changing the stale point of view that this disease is irreversible.

Senile dementia is characterized by numerous disease causes and variability in the conditions associated with this disease. The majority of elderly persons around 65 years of age have numerous types of diseases in their bodies. In addition, their bodies and essence spirit activities, including their brains, have slowly degenerated. Because immunity in the aged has declined, their resistance to disease is already weakened. Again, owing to various diseases, they regularly take different kinds of drugs, but their ability to break down and excrete these drugs' toxins has also been weakened. Thus, chronic drug toxicity is one of the disease causes of this disease. Loneliness and solitude caused by unpleasant emotional experiences in life, such as separation from sons and daughters, bereavement of spouses, and decrease in social activities are internal essence spirit causative factors of this disease. It also sometimes happens that, during acute attack of infectious disease, troubles in consciousness appear and that, when the acute attack is over, senile dementia manifests itself. All these confirm that lack of connection of visceral qi with the brain qi accounts for the disease mechanism of this disease.

Disease causes, disease mechanisms

During old age, qi and blood are deficient and suffer detriment. The construction and defensive are not regulated. The functions of the five viscera lose their harmony, become debilitated and retreat. Therefore, clear yang is not upborne, and turbid yin is not downborne. The spirit brilliance daily suffers detriment. In addition, induced by various evil stimuli, there appear qi stagnation, blood stasis, and phlegm congelation which mist the portals of the heart. Thus qi and blood are not able to fill and nourish the mansion of the original spirit. Rather, they produce bewilderment and chaos in the spiritual mechanism and hence develop into this disease.

Treatment based on pattern discrimination

A. Qi stagnation & blood stasis

Main symptoms: Emotional agitation, worry, and restlessness, irritation, anger, excessive speech, or torpor, stagnation, and scanty speech, eccentric fantasies, chest and lateral costal distention and oppression, a dark, stagnant complexion, a purple tongue with a thin coating, and a wiry, choppy pulse

Treatment principles: Quicken the blood and transform stasis, rectify the qi and resolve depression

Rx: Semen Pruni Persicae (*Tao Ren*), 9g, Radix Rubrus Paeoniae Lactiflorae (*Chi Shao*), 9g, Radix Ligustici Wallichii (*Chuan Xiong*), 9g, Flos Carthami Tinctorii (*Hong Hua*), 9g, Rhizoma Pinelliae Ternatae (*Ban Xia*), 9g, Radix Salviae Miltiorrhizae (*Dan Shen*), 15g, Radix Bupleuri (*Chai Hu*), 6g, Rhizoma Cyperi Rotundi (*Xiang Fu*), 6g, Pericarpium Viridis Citri Reticulatae (*Qing Pi*), 6g, Pericarpium Citri Reticulatae (*Chen Pi*), 6g, Hirudo (*Shui Zhi*), 3g, Rhizoma Acori Graminei (*Chang Pu*), 9g, Tuber Curcumae (*Yu Jin*), 9g

B. Qi vacuity & blood stasis

Main symptoms: All day no speech, no sound, lack of constancy in crying and laughing, no interest in delicious food; on the contrary, the patient may be fond of eating grass and wood. There is also shortness of breath, lack of strength, a lusterless spirit color (*i.e.* complexion), a pale purple tongue, and a fine, choppy pulse

Treatment principles: Boost the qi and upbear yang, quicken the blood and open the portals

Rx: Radix Astragali Membranacei (*Huang Qi*), 15g, Radix Salviae Miltiorrhizae (*Dan Shen*), 15g, Radix Puerariae (*Ge Gen*), 9g, Radix Rubrus Paeoniae Lactiflorae (*Chi Shao*), 9g, Radix Albus Paeoniae

Lactiflorae (*Bai Shao*), 9g, Radix Ligustici Wallichii (*Chuan Xiong*), 9g, Semen Pruni Persicae (*Tao Ren*), 9g, Flos Carthami Tinctorii (*Hong Hua*), 9g, Cortex Phellodendri (*Huang Bai*), 6g, Medulla Tetrapanacis Papyriferi (*Tong Tian Cao*), 9g, Hirudo (*Shui Zhi*), 3g, Fructus Zizyphi Jujubae (*Da Zao*), 5 pieces

C. Phlegm & stasis joining & obstructing

Main symptoms: Emotional tension and agitation, headache, loss of sleep, possible uncontrollable mania, chaotic, rambling talk, anger, unwillingness to live, a purple tongue with a slimy coating, and a wiry, slippery or slippery rapid pulse

Treatment principles: Quicken the blood and transform stasis, break up phlegm and open the portals

Rx: Rhizoma Coptidis Chinensis (*Huang Lian*), 3g, Rhizoma Pinelliae Ternatae (*Ban Xia*), 9g, Concretio Siliceae Bambusae (*Tian Zhu Huang*), 6g, Tuber Curcumae (*Yu Jin*), 9g, Rhizoma Acori Graminei (*Chang Pu*), 9g, bile(-processed) Rhizoma Arisaematis (*Dan Xing*), 9g, Semen Pruni Persicae (*Tao Ren*), 9g, Radix Rubrus Paeoniae Lactiflorae (*Chi Shao*), 9g, Fructus Immaturus Citri Seu Ponciri (*Zhi Shi*), 9g, Medulla Tetrapancis Papyriferi (*Tong Tian Cao*), 9g, Hirudo (*Shui Zhi*), 3g

Secret Essentials

In treating senile dementia, I like to use Hirudo (*Shui Zhi*) to break stasis without damaging qi and blood. If it is combined with Medulla Tetrapanacis Papyriferi (*Tong Tian Cao*), then the light and clear will rise upward, leading the other medicinals to the brain. The treatment effects are marked.

9
Conclusion

For many years, a great number of scholars in our country (*i.e.*, China) have advanced numerous theories on the cause of senility. These have included imbalance of yin and yang, viscera and bowel deficiency and debility, and damage and consumption of essence, qi, and spirit. However, there are few discussions on the influence of the theory of qi and blood on the senility of the organism.

The theory of qi and blood is the core theory of TCM. In terms of basic TCM theory, yin/ yang and five phase theory primarliy serve as systems of philosophical thought, although they have produced a certain influence on the theory of traditional Chinese medicinals. And although the viscera and bowels and channels and network vessels are important constituents in human anatomy and physiology, yet they are by no means the crux in determining the rise, decline, survival, and termination of one's life. Only qi and blood are the most basic substances constituting the human body. They are the material basis for the physiological activities of the tissues and organs, such as the viscera and bowels and channels and network vessels. In the human body, the procession from growth, development, and youthful vigor to senility is but a procession from weakness to strength and from surplus to insufficiency of the qi and blood. The substance of life lies in the qi and blood. Even though in human beings, birth, senility, disease, and death may manifest in numerous forms, yet, in the final analysis, they cannot be separated from changes in the qi and blood. Therefore, the theory of qi and blood is the theoretical basis for my research on combatting senility.

For this reason, I believe that, in combatting senility and conducting research on gerontology, the task of digging out the TCM theories on qi and blood is necessarily of great importance. Through literary and laboratory research plus clinical observation and the employment of modern scientific knowledge and methods, I and my associates are conducting such research on the substance of qi and blood in TCM, and, I further believe that, with the constant elucidation of the substance of qi and blood, the mysteries of human senility will definitely be thoroughly exposed.

Senility and geriatric diseases are mostly characterized by vacuity. Physicians in different dynasties have written numerous dissertations on this point, and this view is generally accepted by people nowadays. However, it should be observed that, with advancing years, because the human body has long been subject to the influence of the six environmental excesses, the seven emotions, food and drink, one's lifestyle, and a variety of diseases, there first appears imbalance in the qi and blood, then obstruction in the movement and transportation of the qi and blood, and eventually engenderment of static blood internally. Owing to the presence of blood stasis, the viscera and bowels cannot obtain nourishment. It is this that leads to imbalance in yin and yang, deficiency and debility in the viscera and bowels, and damage and consumption of essence, qi, and spirit. Thus it is blood stasis which causes the senility of the organism and even death.

Further, it is commonly seen clinical practice that in most geriatric diseases, such as coronary heart disease, cerebral vascular disease, diabetes mellitus, prostatic hyperplasia, and various tumors, there exists the hidden danger of blood stasis. This is so even though the manifestations of these diseases are not all the same. Yet, on examination, the pattern of blood stasis typically can be found playing a role in the disease mechanisms of these geriatric diseases. In that case, supplementing vacuity is simply emphasizing the shadow or surface, while transforming stasis is to really treat the root. Therefore, the theory of blood stasis is fraught with extraordinary significance in the senility of the organism and in preventing and treating geriatric diseases.

I predict that in the future in our country research on combatting senility will clearly reveal the relationship between senility and blood stasis. Thus the theory on senility in Traditional Chinese Medicine will constantly be deepened, forming a new Chinese medical theory on combatting senility and establishing a new school of thought in gerontology. Under the guidance of this new theory and new school of thought, the level of therapeutic efficacy in preventing and treating geriatric diseases will definitely be greatly raised. Not only will it open a new way for treating common geriatric diseases, such as cardiac and cerebral vascular disease and high cholesterol, but it will likewise solve the problem of treating certain recalcitrant geriatric diseases, such as senile dementia and paralysis agitans, for which modern medicine lacks effective therapy or the side effects of the medicinals used are relatively great.

The ancient volumes in TCM have recorded more than 400 kinds of medicinals for combatting senility. For various historical reasons, most physicians have laid undue emphasis on the theory of senility caused by vacuity detriment and on the development of correspondingly supplementing medicinals. Thus research on medicinals for combating senility has developed lop-sidedly. For many years, no satisfactory progress has been made in this respect.

I and my associates have conducted research on combatting senility by developing the therapy of rectifying the qi and quickening the blood. We have scored certain successes by breaking through the theory of vacuity detriment and senility. Our research demonstrates that "balancing yin and yang so as to regulate the qi and blood" is "to strengthen the essence and clear the origin." Clearing the origin is soley in order to strengthen the essence, while strengthening the essence necessarily requires clearing the origin. In other words, this method activates the metabolism, improves physiological and chemical processes, and effectively combats senility and prevents or treats geriatric diseases.

By researching blood stasis and it relationship to the mechanisms of senility and through profound development in the prevention and treatment of geriatric diseases based on that research, we will definitely be able to take a new leap forward in theory and practice. Thus we will contribute towards enriching gerontology and the theory for combatting senility as well as the health and longevity of all humankind.

General Index

A

abdomen and perineum, aching and pain in the lower 236
abdomen, lower, tender, painful, and tense 54
abdomen, lower, tense 125
abdomen, slight discomfort in the 124
abdominal and perineal distention and pain, lower 236
abdominal binding and tension, lower 2402
abdominal cavity, tumor in the 57
abdominal distention 34, 37, 40, 43, 52, 122, 211, 218, 222, 226
abdominal distention, fullness, and oppression 122
abdominal distention, fullness, and tension, lower 52
abdominal distention, fullness, upper 218
abdominal hardness, fullness, and aching, lower 86
abdominal masses 54
abdominal pain, insidious 163
abdominal pain, slight 117
abdominal patterns, acute 87
abdominal region distended, full 54
abdominal wall, engorged vessels on the 218
acne rosacea 53
adnexitis 81
agitation, easy 52, 206
albumin increased 58
alcohol, drinking 56
amenorrhea 37, 55, 72, 73, 86
ancestral qi 11, 12, 19
Ancient & Modern Medicine Gathered Together 193
anger and joy, lack of constancy in 52, 80
anger, easy 52, 56, 82, 134, 135, 141, 144, 198, 203, 206, 240
anger, excessive 153

angina pectoris 81, 100, 107, 189
anuria 225
anus, burning heat around the 118
appendicitis 87
appendix, cystic 86
appetite, devitalized 96, 148, 218, 222
appetite, poor 37, 70, 117, 137, 141, 155, 182, 226
apprehension 51, 203
arcus senilis 67
arteriosclerosis 43, 47, 58, 65, 96, 100, 213
arteriosclerosis, cerebral 43, 58, 65, 100
arthritis, rheumatoid 83
asthma 52, 64, 112, 113, 116
atherosclerosis, coronary artery 183
atony patterns 170
auditory acuity, loss of 134, 135, 140
auditory acuity, episodic loss of 135
auditory acuity, changes in 67
auricles, scorched, dry 195
awoken easily 148

B

back pain extending to the chest, upper 184
balancing method 1, 2, 79, 93, 95, 96, 99, 102, 142, 151, 187 192
Balancing Method #1 93
Balancing Method #2 96
Balancing Method #3 99
Balancing Method #4 102
Balancing Method Sagelike Formula 2, 142, 151, 189, 192
Balancing Method Soluble Preparation 2
baldness 66, 93
bao mai 73
belching 149, 198, 206
Bequeathed Writings on Cautions & Abstentions 36
bi, blood 37, 44, 73

bi, chest 84, 101, 183
bi, cold 166
bi, damp 167
bi, fixed 165, 167
bi, heat 165, 167
bi, painful 165, 166
bi pain of the four limbs 81
bi patterns 62, 164, 165, 170
bi, skin 207
bi, wind 166
bi zheng 164
bilirubin, high 57
Bing Ji Sha Zhuang 16
bladder heat 125
bladder, stasis obstructing the 236
bleeding from the flesh 50
bleeding patterns 21, 23, 60, 64, 66, 72, 160, 161, 164, 220
bleeding, upper digestive tract 88
bleeding, uterine 34, 42, 44, 45, 50, 55
blindness 67
blockage pattern 188, 189
blockage, yang 188, 189
blockage, yin 188
blood, accumulated 46
blood, coagulated 46
blood clots 40, 55, 127
blood counterflow 36, 40-42, 188
blood, dark but pale 163
blood, dead 46
blood desertion 24, 36, 44, 45
blood, dry 45, 68, 159
blood, foul 46
blood heat 82, 213, 224
blood leaving the channel 46
blood, malign 45, 215
blood, retained 45, 46
blood rheology 47, 56, 93, 94, 96
blood, routine examination of the 58
blood sedimentation 58
blood stasis 1, 10, 20, 31, 33, 35-40, 42, 47, 55, 59-61, 64-69, 72, 85, 97, 98, 106, 107, 130, 133, 142, 154, 158, 162, 188, 191, 192, 198, 207, 211, 215-218, 221-223, 228, 231, 234, 235, 237, 239-242, 244, 245, 248-250
blood stasis & qi stagnation 212
blood stasis internally stopped 158
blood, vacuity not containing 163
bodily heaviness 109, 117, 185
body and limbs, aching and pain 43
body, cold 119
body, heavy 170
bowel movement per week, one 124
bradycardia 100
breath, bad 122, 188
breath, shortness of 34, 37, 38, 44, 64, 89, 96, 114, 115, 123, 156, 184-186, 205, 223, 231, 245
breathing, distressed rapid dyspneic 156
breathing, faint 189
breathing, forceful 188, 230
breathing, hard 176
breathing, movement stirs rapid 181
bronchiectasis 82
bronchitis, chronic 65, 96
bronchitis, senile 84
burping, frequent 123

C

cachectic diseases 90
cancer 43, 215
cancer, liver 215
capillary loops, abnormal 56
cardiac motion 57
cardiac infarction, painless 193
cardiac rhythm, irregular 100
cardiac ventricle hypertrophic 57
cardiopulmonary disease 43
cataracts, senile 67
central qi insufficiency 136
cerebral arteriosclerosis 43, 58, 65, 100
cerebral stroke 187, 191
cerebral vascular disease, occlusive 99, 100
cerebral vessels, insufficient blood supply to the 96

Chao Shi Bing Yuan 125
Chao Yuan-fang 45
cheeks of the face, water swelling of 222
cheeks are flushed red 53, 158
cheeks, dilation of capillaries on the nail bed and 69
chest and abdomen, chilly pain in 81
chest and lateral costal aching and pain 80
chest and lateral costal glomus and fullness 198
chest and lateral costal radiating pain 162
chest *bi* 84, 101, 183
chest, insidious, burning pain 90
chest oppression, fullness 43, 96, 101, 113, 117, 135, 153, 182, 185, 199, 203, 206, 229
chest, blockage and oppression within 184
chest pain 84, 96, 101, 147, 175, 176, 183, 185
chest pain with cough and phlegm mixed with 84
chest yang *bi* & obstruction 184
chill 121, 122, 124, 156, 168, 175, 177, 186, 205, 223
chill, dread of 205
chin, dark color below the 53
cholecystitis 40, 87
cholelithiasis 40, 87
chong and *ren* 73, 197
chyle in the serum 58
Classic of Difficulties 8, 122
climacteric syndrome, female 201, 206
climacteric syndrome, male 204
clots 38, 40, 50, 55, 127
cold and heat, alternating 49
cold, aversion to 109, 143, 166, 176, 222
cold, common 108, 110-112
cold, damage 109, 175
cold, fear of 108, 113, 155, 186, 199, 205, 223, 231

cold, sometimes hot, sometimes 203
colitis, chronic 80
coma, hypertonic 193
complexion, bloodless white 163
complexion, bright white 205
complexion, clear, white 124
complexion, dark, black 136, 195
complexion, dark, stagnant 145, 245
complexion, flushed red 156
complexion, lusterless 44, 123, 140, 144, 152, 226
complexion, poor 96
complexion, sallow yellow 37, 119, 155, 222
complexion, scant luster to the facial 148
complexion, somber, dark 155, 2253 231
complexion, somber white 45, 131, 177, 186
complexion, somber, white, lusterless 44
constipation 52, 86, 121-124, 135, 144, 162, 180, 188, 198, 203, 217, 240
constipation, chill 121, 122, 124
constipation, dry heat 122
constipation, qi stagnation & vacuity 123
constipation, senile habitual 124
constitution, weak 140
constructive qi 11, 13, 23
contagious qi 56
coolness, desire for, and aversion to heat 171
corneal diseases 67
coronary artery atherosclerosis 183
Correction of Errors in the Medical Forest 40
costal regions, bilateral insidious pain in the lateral 216
cough 34, 43, 52, 64, 84, 96, 108-110, 112-116, 157, 161, 175, 176, 177, 227-231
cough and abundant phlegm 113
cough and asthma 64

cough and wheezing 114, 116
cough, bloody 156
cough, loud 108
cough, phlegmy 43
cough, spasmodic 161
cough with itchy throat 109
cough with yellow phlegm 110
coughing sound, low, weak 114
counterflow and chaos of the qi and
    blood 41
crying and scolding, incessant 240
cyanosis 62, 64, 69

D

damp heat & stasis binding 217, 236
dampness causing blood stasis 216
Dan Xi Xin Fa 64
Dan-xi's Heart Methods 64
deafness 34, 67, 133-138
deafness as if obstructed 136
deafness, sudden 134
defecate, willingness to yet no force
    to do so 123
defecation, inhibited 149
defecation not easy 123
defensive qi 9, 11, 14, 109, 147, 229
dementia, senile 47, 60, 85, 243, 244,
    246, 249
desertion pattern 45, 189
*Detailed Outline of the Study of
    Medicine* 233
diabetes mellitus 90, 192, 193, 195,
    196, 248
diabetic renal diseases 193
diarrhea 38, 52, 116-121, 202, 222
diarrhea, cold damp 117
diarrhea, damp heat 118
diarrhea, fifth watch *i.e.*, daybreak
    119
diarrhea, kidney vacuity 119
diarrhea, spleen vacuity 118
diarrhea with untransformed grain
    119
digestive tract bleeding, upper 88

*Direct Formulas from the Study of
    Mercy* 108
Disease Mechanism Sand Seal 16
disease, slow onset of 171
diverticula 57
dizziness 37, 43, 45, 65, 66, 93, 96,
    123, 128, 131, 132, 134,
    137-142, 144, 148, 155, 161,
    163, 171, 179-182, 185, 203-206,
    222
dizziness and vertigo 37, 65, 131,
    137, 142
dizziness inversion 45
Dong Yuan Shi Shu 62
dreams, chaotic 241
dreams, excessive 34, 43, 51, 65, 80,
    148, 149, 157, 181
dreams which are filled with fright,
    apprehension, and 51
dribbling and dripping 44, 125, 127,
    177, 186, 235, 237
drool flows by itself 191
drum distention 215, 216
Du Yi Sui Bi 12, 23
dumbness disease 187
dysmenorrhea 55, 81
dyspnea and cough 175

E

ear wax mixed with old blood 136
eating grass and wood, fond of 245
eczema, skin 222
edema 54, 65, 71, 96, 113, 205, 218,
    220, 221, 223, 225, 229, 231
edema, pitting 221, 223
edema, superficial 55, 96, 113, 205,
    218, 220, 221, 225, 229, 231
edema, superficial, marked below the
    waist 225
edema, superficial, of the entire body
    229
edema, superficial, of the eyelids 221
edema, superficial, of the lower limbs
    55, 218, 229
ejaculate, failure to 104

ejaculation, premature 102, 104, 131, 137, 148, 155, 171, 195, 205
electrocardiogram 57, 99
emaciation, bodily 114, 194
emotional depression 34, 52, 80, 93, 183, 193, 207
emotional tension, agitation 214, 246
emphysema 64, 65
Entering the Gate of the Study of Medicine 73
epigastric and abdominal aching and pain 52
epigastric and abdominal distention and falling 222
epigastric and abdominal glomus and pain 162
epigastric oppression, distention, and fullness 149
epigastric pain and burning heat 162
epilepsy 56, 58, 84
epistaxis 42, 45, 50, 88, 161
erection during intercourse, lack of 130, 131
eructations, acid 198
essence spirit bitter and oppressed 131
essence blood deficiency detriment 137
essence, deficiency and consumption of the 47
essence spirit abstraction 242
essence spirit, devitalized 113, 155
essence spirit withering and wilting 131, 140
essence spirit worry and depression 205, 235
Essentials from the Golden Cabinet 37, 44, 45, 139, 220
external injury 50, 56, 83, 145
external injury, history of 56, 145
eyes dark and blackish 158
eyes, darkening of 163
eyes, red 144, 162, 180
eyesight, decline in 67

F

face may be bluish purple 53
face, red 135, 162, 180, 203, 240
face and eyes, red 203, 240
face, red, hot 144
falling and fainting, sudden 241
fantasies, eccentric 245
fatigue 34, 37, 38, 44, 70, 93, 109, 114, 117, 118, 136, 139, 144, 147, 148, 154, 163, 177, 186, 197, 218, 220, 222, 223, 242
fatigue, spiritual 44, 114, 118, 136, 144, 148, 163, 177, 186, 218, 223
fear, easy 131, 152
feces are yellowish brown 118
feet atonic and weak 157
fever 49, 50, 93, 108-111, 134, 156, 162, 166, 170, 175, 176-178, 203, 205, 222
fever but no cold 176
fever, high 49, 175, 178
fever, low 177
fever, localized 49
fever, night 203
fever, periodic 49
fever, tidal 49, 93, 156, 161, 204
fever, tidal, in the afternoon 49
fingers and toes are enlarged, ends of the 55
fingers, trembling 226
five hearts, vexatious heat in 90, 148, 181
flatulence, foul-smelling 199
fluids and humors 7, 8, 12, 13, 15, 17, 18, 23, 42, 43, 71, 112, 122, 124, 234
food or drink, no thought for 163, 206
foods, eating sweet, fatty 56
foot weakness, low back soreness and 186
fright and fear 131
fright palpitations 157
fright, susceptibility to 152

frightened, easily 147, 149, 203, 242
frigidity, female 103

G

gastritis, chronic 40, 196
General Collection for Holy Relief 63
genitalia, atrophy of the 102
geriatric diseases 39, 43, 47, 96, 103, 105-107, 175, 248-250
goiter 85
Gu Jin Yi Jian 69
Gu Jin Yi Tong 193
Guidebook to Clinical Patterns 197
gum redness and swelling 226
gums, bleeding 161, 162
gynecological diseases 81

H

hair, postpartum falling of 55
hair is withered and dry 52
hands and feet clear, chilly 118-119
hands and feet, lack of warmth in the 124
hands spread open 189
head distention 139, 141
head, heavy, as if covered 140
head with a scarf, fondness for covering one's 144
headache 43, 95, 108-110, 134, 135, 139, 141-146, 162, 180-182, 221, 222, 226, 246
headache, blood vacuity 144
headache, liver yang 144
headache, obstinate 146
headache, persistent 145
headache radiating to the nape of the neck 143
headache, static blood 145
headache, wind cold 143
heart and chest piercing pain 184
heart arrhythmia 99
heart blood deficiency & vacuity 203
heart disease, coronary 43, 80, 85, 89, 99, 100, 183, 187, 248

heart loss of nourishment 152
heart may be enlarged 57
heart pain 52, 60-62, 183-187
heart pain, inversion 183
heart pain, true 183
heart pain radiating to the upper back 184
heart palpitations 21, 34, 37, 43, 52, 60-62, 64, 96, 123, 131, 144, 147-149, 151, 152, 163, 180-182, 185, 186, 203, 223, 242
heart palpitations and throbbing 186
heart, phlegm stasis confounding the 231
heart, paroxysmal auricular premature beat of 99
heart, paroxysmal ventricular premature beat of 99
heart qi insufficiency 62, 100
heart, racing 60-62, 90, 144, 151-153, 157
heart, racing with perspiration 152
heart skipping 147
heart spirit 20, 34, 202
heart spirit bewildered & chaotic 202
heart/spleen insufficiency 148
heart vessel stasis & obstruction 184
heart vexation 51, 118, 131, 135, 144, 148, 149, 157, 177, 184, 203, 235, 241
heat, an abnormal feeling of 150, 153
heat brewing & forcing the blood 162
heat, sudden feelings of 205
heel pain 237
hemafecia 42, 50, 160
hematuria 44, 50, 162
hemiplegia 62, 63, 86, 88, 187, 188, 190, 192
hemoptysis 42, 50, 52, 88
hemorrhage 18, 20, 24, 41, 44, 45, 163, 190, 215, 221
hemorrhagic diseases 44, 88, 164
heng fa 1, 2, 93-99, 102, 142, 151, 187, 192
Heng Fa Chong Ji 2

Heng Fa Er Hao 96-98
Heng Fa San Hao 99
Heng Fa Sheng Fang 2, 142, 151, 187, 192
Heng Fa Si Hao 102
Heng Fa Yi Hao 93-97, 99, 102
hepatic and biliary systems, diseases of the 80
hepatitis 40, 82, 89, 215, 216, 219
hepatitis, chronic 40, 89, 215, 216
hepatomegaly 86
herpes zoster 209
hot flashes 93
Huang Di Nei Jing 3
Huang Han Yi Xue 67
hunger, easy 194
hyperlipidemia 57, 84, 96
hypertension 47, 84, 85, 96, 179, 188, 221
hypochondral region, fullness and oppression in the 123
hysteria 80, 93

I

impotence 72, 73, 102, 104, 130-133, 137, 154, 155, 171, 195
impotence, senile 104
infertility, female 55, 81
infertility, male 55
insomnia 34, 51, 80, 93, 95, 96, 144, 147-151, 180, 185
intelligence, diminished 59, 60
intestinal rumbling 119
intestines and stomach, accumulation of heat in 122
intestines, scanty fluids, moisture 121
itching 50, 134, 170, 195, 213-215, 222, 226
itching, ceaseless 222
itching occurs spasmodically 50

J

jaundice which does not recede 52

jealousy, excessive 52
Jin Gui Yao Lue 37, 44, 45, 70, 139, 192, 220, 227
Jing Yue Quan Shu 16, 29, 42, 117, 160, 196
joint soreness and pain 134
joints cannot bend or stretch 51
joints of the four limbs, aching and pain of the 83
joints, pain in the 83
jue yin 142, 146

K

Keeping the Flame of the Lamp of Medicine Lit 65
kidney essence deficiency detriment 131
kidney essence insufficiency 140
kidney qi deficiency & vacuity 195
kidney vacuity 1, 72, 103, 119, 125
kidney yang vacuity & debility 154-155
kidney yang vacuity weakness 186
kidney yin & yang dual vacuity 205

L

lateral costal fullness 153
lateral costal region, insidious pain in 216
Law in Medical Science 69
Lei Jing 26
leukemia 90
Li Dong-yuan 13
light, fear of 205
limb and body aching and pain 73
limb atony and weakness, lower 171
limbs and body, atonic, weak, forceless 171
limbs, atony and weakness of the four 172
limbs, body, and joints, soreness and pain of the 166

limbs, chilled 101, 119, 137, 155, 189, 202
limbs, inability to use the 63
limbs, inversion chill of the four 177, 186, 223
Lin Zheng Zhi Nan 196
lines, thin, red 53
Ling Shu 5, 9, 16, 17, 25, 27-29, 39, 42, 59, 61, 66, 68, 75, 77, 78, 133, 196, 215, 219, 227
lips and nails are purple 229
lips and nails, bluish purple 38, 223
lips and nails, lusterless 37, 137
lips, blue face and purple 101
lips, bluish purple 38, 223, 241
lips, cyanotic 65
Liu Wan-su 193
live, unwillingness to 246
liver blood stasis & obstruction 217
liver cancer 215
liver, cirrhosis of the 89, 90, 107, 215
liver fire counterflows upward 180
liver fire mixed with stasis 198, 240
liver/gallbladder depressive fire 210
liver/gallbladder fire exuberance 135
liver/kidney deficiency & vacuity 171
liver/kidney essence vacuity 157
liver qi depression and accumulation 80
liver wind 141, 179, 180, 226
liver wind internally stirring 226
liver yang 139, 143, 144, 179, 188
liver yang hyperactive above 139
liver, worry and anxiety damaging the 130
low back pain, wringing 126
low back and knee chilly pain 237
low back and knee soreness and weakness 119, 126, 128, 131, 140, 181, 195, 205, 225
low back chill 155
low back soreness 34, 131, 137, 157, 186

low back soreness and foot weakness 186
low back, knee, and feet weakness 181
lower and upper back chill and heaviness 124
lumbar muscle taxation and detriment 83
lumps, swollen 43, 54, 55
lung abscess 82, 84
lung distention 175, 227-229
lung defensive, evils assailing 176
lung heat, fluids damaged 193
lung/stomach fluid vacuity 156
lungs, phlegm heat congesting the 176
lungs, tumor in the 57
lupus cells 58

M

Ma Yuan-yi 154
Mai Yi Zheng Zhi 215
mania and withdrawl 238
Master Chao's Origins of Disease 125
Master Shen's Book on Respecting Life 220
Master Zhang's Medical Knowledge 17, 65
memory, diminished force of 205
memory, poor 34, 43, 51, 59, 60, 93, 141, 148, 157, 180, 181, 205
menopausal syndrome 56, 93
menopause 56, 201, 202
menstrual pain 81
menstruation, delayed 37, 155
menstruation, irregular 55
menstruation, scanty 37, 40, 55
mental diseases 56
mental dullness 241
ministerial fire 42, 133, 161
ministerial fire, effulgent 133
moles, black 55
mouth and tongue, sores on the 157

mouth, bitter taste in the 135, 139, 144, 180, 198, 203, 222
mouth, dry 51, 110, 161, 176, 185, 194, 195, 203, 222
mouth, dry, and thirst 110
mouth, dry, leading to drinking 176
mouth, dry with scant fluids 185
mouth, pasty slime within the 185
mouth, slimy, and sweet taste 226
mouth, wry 63
myasthenia gravis 170

N

nail bed microcirculation 56, 96
nails are bluish purple 54, 186
Nan Jing 8, 22
nausea 52, 138, 140, 182, 225, 226
navel bulges out 54
neoplastic tissue 69
nervous diseases, functional 80
nervous tension 179, 203
neurasthenia 40, 93, 94
night sweats 156, 205
nightmare 93, 150
nose heat 162
nose, runny 108, 109
nose, stuffy 109, 110
nose, stuffy, with turbid discharge 110
nostrils, flaring 176
Notes on the Study of Medicine 12, 23, 73
numbness 34, 37, 51, 73, 171, 172, 180, 190
numbness and insensitivity 172
numbness in the four limbs 180
numbness, muscle and skin 73

O

oral ulcers 226
original qi 11, 38, 45, 74, 112, 154, 177
original qi vacuity desertion 177

Orthodox Ancestral External Medicine 210
ovarian cysts 86

P

pain and urgency, piercing 126
pain, chilly feeling at the place of 166
pain exacerbated by exposure to wind and cold 143
pain fixed in a certain spot 145
pain, fixed, stable, which refuses pressure 198
pain, generalized 109
pain in the chest and lateral costal regions 79
pain in the chest, lateral costal regions 82, 90
pain in the heart and abdomen 81
pain, intense, aching and 168
pain made worse by pressure 50
pain, light in the day, more severe at night 166
pain, local 49
pain mild in the day and severe at night 199
pain, obstructive 81
pain, pricking 125, 127, 199
pain which refuses pressure, very intense 198
palpitations 21, 34, 37, 43, 45, 51, 52, 60-62, 64, 96, 123, 131, 144, 147-149, 151, 152, 157, 163, 180-182, 185, 186, 203, 223, 242
palpitations, fright 157
Pan Ji 65
pancreatitis 87
panting 12, 34, 43, 52, 64, 112-115, 227, 229-231
panting, enduring 52
paralysis 84, 170, 251
paralysis, periodic 170
patches, darkish, brown 52
Patches, large whitish or atrophic, 67
patches, longevity 68

patches, old age 68
patches, purplish 55
patches, static 53, 55, 114, 141, 145, 166, 184, 212, 222, 236
pattern discrimination based on channel differentiation 142
Patterns, Causes, Pulses & Treatment 63
pelvic inflammation, chronic 86
penis is not hard 130
penis, pain in the 235
perspiration 101, 109, 121, 122, 147, 152, 177, 185, 186, 202
perspiration, daybreak 147
perspiration, excessive 122
perspiration, great 177, 186
perspiration, no 109
perspiration, spontaneous 177, 185, 203
phlebitis 90
phlegm 2, 30, 33-36, 42, 43, 46, 52, 54, 63-65, 80, 84-86, 98, 100, 101, 109, 110, 112-116, 134-136, 139-143, 162, 175, 176, 177, 179, 182, 183, 185, 188-191, 199, 228-232, 241, 242, 244, 246
phlegm & stasis binding together 199
phlegm & stasis joining & binding 241
phlegm & stasis joining & obstructing 246
phlegm and stasis 2, 36, 42, 43, 85, 115
phlegm, bloody 52
phlegm dampness 134, 143, 182
phlegm dampness congestion & exuberance 182
phlegm, excessive, like white froth 229
phlegm, excessive, watery, thin 109
phlegm, extremely excessive 185
phlegm fire depression & binding 135
phlegm heat mixed with stasis 230
phlegm like white foam 115
phlegm nodulations 54, 85

phlegm obstruction 42, 63-65
phlegm, red-looking 161
phlegm rheum 112-116, 139
phlegm, spitting out rusty colored 175
phlegm stasis congesting the lungs 229
phlegm streaked with red 52
phlegm turbidity 30, 33-35, 43, 46, 64, 140, 179, 183, 185
phlegm turbidity internally obstructing 185
phlegm turbidity obstructing the center 140
phlegm which is watery, white colored 113
phlegm, yellow or white, which is pasty 230
phlegm, yellow, pasty 176
Pi Wei Lun 13, 26
plaques, senile 47
pneumonia 107, 175, 178
pneumonia, lobar 175
polydipsia 192, 194
polyneuritis 170
polyphagia 192, 194
polyps 57
polyuria 125, 192, 235
porphyria 81
positive rheumatoid factors 58
postpartum falling of hair 55
postpartum lochia which will not stop 55
postpartum uterine bleeding 55
pregnancy, ectopic 81, 87
progressive muscular dystrophy 170
prostatic hyperplasia 47, 72, 232, 233, 235, 248
prostatic hypertrophy 86, 96, 233
pruritus, senile 213
pulmonary heart disease 65, 107, 227-229, 232
pulmonary heart disease, chronic 227, 232
pyorrhea 50

Q

qi & yin dual deficiency 185
qi & yin dual vacuity 177
qi counterflow 36, 40-42, 69, 142, 162
qi counterflow damaging the network vessels 161
qi desertion 36, 44, 45
qi mechanism is depressed and stagnant 122
qi stagnation & blood stasis 39, 235, 241, 245
qi stagnation, blood stasis 198, 244
qi transformation 4, 6-8, 15, 18, 30, 71, 221, 223, 225, 234, 237, 238
qi vacuity & blood stasis 37, 218, 222, 242, 245

R

Raynaud's disease 81
ren mai 21
Ren Zhao Zhi Zhi Fang 108
reproductive abnormality 55
respiration, rapid 115
respiratory failure 229
rheoencephalography 57
rheum, sticky, pasty 112
rheumatoid arthritis 83

S

sadness is so damaging one feels like weeping 202
san bao 25
scars, red 53
sciatica 83
sclera are static and turbid 53
sclera may also be tinged yellow 53
scleroderma 107, 207, 209
sclerotic opacities 47
scrofula 54, 85
senility, premature 96, 102, 103
septicemia 82

sexual function, decline in the male's 102
sexual function, diminished 72, 130, 205
sexual troubles, male 103
shang han 60, 175, 239
Shang Han Lun 60, 239
shao yang 142, 146
shao yin 61, 66, 142, 146
Shen Jin-ao 101
Shen Zhai Yi Su 36
Sheng Ji Zong Lu 63
shivering, cold 176
shou ban 68
Shou Shi Bai Yuan (Protecting the Origin of Longevity) 196
shoulder, periarthritis of the 83
sighs, heaving 203
Simple Questions 3, 5, 6, 12, 16-18, 21, 23, 28-33, 35, 39, 41, 61-63, 71-73, 75-77, 106, 233, 240
sinew atony 130, 170
sinews and vessels are stiff and tense 167
sinews, greenish blue 54, 55, 65, 69, 70, 153
skin, bluish purple 172
skin, brown patches on the 68
skin is scaly and dry 55
skin itching 195, 226
skin pigmentation 47
skin, rough 47, 158
skin, scaly, dry 68, 69, 90
sleep at night not tranquil 152
sleep, excessive 140
sleep, loss of 132, 141, 144, 149, 157, 181, 205, 241, 246
sleep not quiet 135, 149
sleep, scanty 65, 66, 90, 139, 153, 203
smoking 55, 212, 214
sneezing 108, 109
speak, inability to 63
speech, disordered 241
speech is not clear 191
speech, raving 51

spermatorrhea 148, 157
spirit, lack of 242
spirit manner rigid and wooden 192
spirit orientation confusion and chaos
51
spiritual fatigue 44, 114, 118, 136,
144, 148, 163, 177, 186, 218,
223
Spiritual Pivot 5, 9, 16, 17, 25,
27-29, 39, 42, 59, 61, 66, 68, 75,
77, 78, 133, 196, 215, 219, 227
spleen/kidney yang vacuity 224, 225
spleen/stomach vacuity cold 155
splenomegaly 86
stasis & heat struggling & binding
221
stasis in the blood mansion 147, 152
stasis obstructing the ancestral vessel
136
stasis obstructing the channels &
vessels 141
stasis obstruction of the vessels &
network vessels 172
static blood 30, 33, 35, 36, 38, 39,
43, 45-49, 55-60, 62, 63, 65-73,
79, 86, 90, 97, 100, 101, 107,
108, 117, 139, 142, 145, 147,
152, 155, 162, 164, 182, 196,
197, 215, 220, 228, 229, 233,
234, 239, 243, 248
stiffness 51
stomach and epigastric burning heat
and piercing pain 198
stomach and epigastric distention and
pain 198
stomach and epigastric intense,
colicky pain 199
stomach and epigastric pricking pain
199
stomach heat intense & exuberant
194
stomach pain 196, 201
stool is thin and loose 116
stool is watery 116
stool, bloody 45
stools, bloody, like lacquer 88

stools, clear, watery 117
stools, dry, bound 230, 236
stools, loose 37, 136, 155, 202, 205,
216, 217
stools precipitating fresh red blood
162
strangury 125-130, 234
strangury, blood 125, 127
strangury, five types of 125
strangury, qi 125-127
strangury, stone 125, 126, 129
strangury, taxation 125, 126, 128
strength, lack of 44, 71, 89, 128, 136,
144, 148, 155, 163, 185, 218,
220, 245
stroke, cerebral 187, 191
stroke, death 187
stroke, sequelae of wind 89, 96, 194
Su Wen 3, 5, 6, 12, 16-18, 21, 23,
28-33, 35, 39, 41, 59, 61-63,
71-73, 75-77, 106, 233, 240
sublingual varices 69
superfluous substance 69
surgery 55
suspicion, excessive 52, 80, 203
sweat, dripping 163
sweat like oil 190
sweats, night 157, 204
sweating 34, 45, 123, 166, 205
swelling and distention 167
syncope 35, 45, 180, 226
Systematized Classic 26

T

tachycardia 100
tai chong mai 21
tai yang 61, 71, 142, 146, 239
tai yin 12, 143, 146
talk, chaotic, rambling 246
talk, disinclination to 38, 44
Tang Rong-chuan 46, 60, 64, 72
taste, no 202
taxation beyond limit 122, 188, 216
Ten Books of Dong-yuan 62
tenesmus 155

terminal dribbling 126, 127, 235
testicles, pain radiating to the 236
The Complete Writings of Jing-yue 15, 16, 29, 117, 160, 196
The Study of imperial Han Medicine 67
The Treatment of Patterns Based on the Pulse 215
The True Understanding of Medical Theory 69
thinking may be confused and chaotic 51
thirst 44, 50, 110, 117, 118, 122, 162, 176, 192, 194, 217, 230
thirst, no 117
thirst, oral 118, 162, 176, 217, 230
thirst, oral, but no desire to drink 217
thirst, oral, leading to drinking 162
throat and mouth, dry 144
throat, dry 52, 135, 144, 157, 163, 199
throat, itchy 108, 109
throat, obstructed sensation in the 241
throat pain 157
throat, phlegmy sounds in the 241
throat, red, swollen, aching and painful 110
throat, sore 108
timidity and excessive suspicions 130
tinnitus 34, 67, 68, 133-139, 148, 152, 157, 163, 180, 181, 205
tinnitus like the chirping of cicadas 134, 136
tinnitus, sudden 134
tomography, computer-assisted 57
torpid intake 211
tranquility, lack of 147, 151
treasures, three 25
Treatise on Bleeding Patterns 21, 23, 60, 64, 66, 72, 222
Treatise on Damage Due to Cold 60, 239
Treatise on the Origins & Symptoms of Various Diseases 26, 193

Treatise on the Spleen & Stomach 13, 26
tremors, convulsive, of the limbs and body 192
triple burner, turbidity flooding the 226
tuberculosis 90
tumor in the abdominal cavity 57
tumors, static 54
tumors, vascular 86

U

ulcerative diseases 89
ulcers 57, 226
ultrasound examination 57
unconsciousness 63
uremia 221, 224, 227, 235
urinary block, dribbling 71, 233, 234
urinary blockage 226
urinary pain 236
urinary retention 144, 188
urinary urgency 236
urinate, constant feeling of the need 236
urinate completely, unable to 125
urinating drop by drop 236
urinating, piercing pain when 162
urination, astringent, painful 127
urination clear and long 124
urination, endless dribbling 129
urination, fine, thready 236
urination, hot, astringent, with pricking pain 127
urination, inhibited 127, 222, 224, 233
urination, interrupted 52
urination is short and red 118, 122, 162
urination, red, astringent 171, 217
urination, scanty 52, 218, 225
urination, short, scanty 218
urination sometimes astringent and painful 52
urination, spontaneous 190
urine, cloudy, turbid 128

urine, deep yellow 222
urine, lack of force in expelling 237
urine mixed with gravel and stones 126
urine, purplish 127
urine, red 203
urine, retention of 72, 233
urine, turbid 52, 128, 195
urine, turbid, like fat or grease 195
urine, turbid, cloudy 236
urine, yellow 176, 222
uterine bleeding 34, 42, 44, 45, 50, 55
uterine bleeding, postpartum 55
uterine fibroids 86

V

vacuity taxation 37, 44, 68, 154, 159, 219
varicose phenomena 69
vasography 57
vertebrae disease, cervical 43
vertebrae, hypertrophy of the cervical 83
vertigo 37, 65, 66, 123, 131, 137-142, 148, 155, 171, 179, 180, 205
vessels, decrease in elasticity of the 70
vexation and agitation 50, 93, 134, 141, 157, 180, 198, 201, 203, 230, 231
vexation, easy 52
violence, easy 52
visceral agitation 201
vision, blurred 152, 205
visual or auditory hallucinations 51
visual power, diminished 67
voice, loss of 156
vomiting large amounts of blood 162
vomiting of phlegmy fluids 182
vomiting white froth 241

W

Wai Ke Zheng Zong 210
Wang Chong 66
Wang Jie-zhai 42
Wang Ken-tang 46
Wang Qing-ren 38, 76, 239
warm disease 175
wasting, lower 195
wasting, middle 194
wasting, upper 193
water blisters 209, 210
water qi disease 223
water swelling 65, 71, 72, 219-222
water swelling of the cheeks of the face 222
weakness, spleen qi vacuity 43, 44
wei zheng 169
wen bing 175
wheezing, movement results in panting and 229
wind and fire fan each other 180
wind, aversion 110, 134
wind cold 108, 109, 113, 143, 175
wind evils externally invading 134
wind, fear of 143, 165
wind heat 108-110, 142, 210
wind stroke 42, 47, 62, 63, 84, 85, 89, 96, 141, 180, 187, 191, 193

X, Y, Z

Xue Zheng Lun 21, 23, 60, 64, 66, 71, 72, 220
yang ming 12, 71, 142, 146, 173
yang sheng 1
yang vacuity & blood stasis 223, 231, 237
yang vacuity tending to desertion 186
yawning, frequent 202
Yellow Emperor's Inner Classic 3
Yi Deng Xu Yan 65
Yi Lin Gai Cuo 40, 60, 65, 66, 68, 70, 94
Yi Meng Fa Lu 69
Yi Xue Gang Mu 233

Yi Xue Ru Men 73
Yi Xue Zheng Chuan 69
yin deficiency, fire effulgence 148
yin vacuity, internal heat 204
yin vacuity, yang hyperactivity 181
yu xue 45, 90
Zhang Jie-bin 15
Zhang Jie-gu 121
Zhang Jing-yue 46, 233
Zhang Shi Yi Tong 17, 65
Zhang Zhong-jing 45, 112, 233
Zheng Yin Mai Zhi 62
Zheng Zhi Hui Bu 220
Zhou Xue-hai 12
Zhu Bing Yuan Hou Lun 26, 69, 192
Zhu Dan-xi 46, 139, 220, 228

About the Author

Prof. Yan De-xin has practiced medicine for over 50 years. Like many Chinese doctors of his generation, Prof. Yan began his study of Chinese medicine while still quite young with his father, Yan Yi-lu, a famous practitioner of Traditional Chinese Medicine. Later, Prof. Yan graduated from the Shanghai College of Traditional Chinese Medicine. Currently, Dr. Yan is a professor at the Shanghai Railway Medical College where he is chief of the TCM Research Section as well as chief physician at the Railway Central Hospital.

Among his many professional credits, Prof. Yan is a Fellow of the Chinese Academy of Integrated Chinese-Western Medicine and a Fellow of the Chinese National Academy of TCM. He is also a specialist member of the Shanghai Academy of TCM and a member of the Council for Determining High Posts in the Health Section of the National Railway Department. He has also been chief of the TCM Specialists Group, a member of the National Council for Determining Prizes in Scientific and Technical Progress in TCM, clinical chief and member on the Shanghai Scientific and Medical Specialists Committee, and chief member of the National Railway TCM Academic Committee. In addition, Prof. Yan has won several academic awards for his special theories and treatments in TCM geriatrics.

Prof. Yan has published hundreds of articles in Chinese TCM journals and is author of a number of books on TCM geriatrics and blood stasis. Translated into English, some of the titles of these are: *Quickening the Blood & Transforming Stasis in Clinical Practice; Qi, Blood & Longevity;* and *Essential Secrets of Combating Senility with TCM* in China through various Dynasties. In short, Prof. Yan is not only one of the most famous TCM geriatric specialists in China, but is regarded as one of China's premier *lao yi sheng* or old masters of medicine. Blue Poppy Press is honored to be able to share his special insights into the TCM treatment of older patients with English readers around the world.

ACUPOINT POCKET REFERENCE by Bob Flaws
ISBN 0-936185-93-7
ISBN 978-0-936185-93-4

ACUPUNCTURE, CHINESE MEDICINE & HEALTHY
WEIGHT LOSS   Revised Edition
by Juliette Aiyana, L. Ac.
ISBN 1-891845-61-6
ISBN 978-1-891845-61-1

ACUPUNCTURE & IVF by Lifang Liang
ISBN 0-891845-24-1
ISBN 978-0-891845-24-6

ACUPUNCTURE FOR STROKE REHABILITATION
Three Decades of Information from China
by Hoy Ping Yee Chan, et al.
ISBN 1-891845-35-7
ISBN 978-1-891845-35-2

ACUPUNCTURE PHYSICAL MEDICINE: An
Acupuncture Touchpoint Approach to the Treatment of
Chronic Pain, Fatigue, and Stress Disorders
by Mark Seem
ISBN 1-891845-13-6
ISBN 978-1-891845-13-0

ACUPUNCTURE MEDICINE: Bodymind Integration
for Bodily Distress and Mental Pain by Mark Seem
ISBN 1-891845-70-5
ISBN 978-1-891845-70-3

AGING & BLOOD STASIS: A New Approach to TCM
Geriatrics by Yan De-xin
ISBN 0-936185-63-6
ISBN 978-0-936185-63-7

AN ACUPUNCTURISTS GUIDE TO MEDICAL RED
FLAGS & REFERRALS by Dr. David Anzaldua, MD
ISBN 1-891845-54-3
ISBN 978-1-891845-54-3

BETTER BREAST HEALTH NATURALLY with
CHINESE MEDICINE
by Honora Lee Wolfe & Bob Flaws
ISBN 0-936185-90-2
ISBN 978-0-936185-90-3

BIOMEDICINE: A TEXTBOOK FOR PRACTITIONERS
OF ACUPUNCTURE AND ORIENTAL MEDICINE by
Bruce H. Robinson, MD Second Edition
ISBN 1-891845-62-4
ISBN 978-1-891845-62-8

THE BOOK OF JOOK: Chinese Medicinal Porridges
by Bob Flaws
ISBN 0-936185-60-6
ISBN 978-0-936185-60-0

CHANNEL DIVERGENCES Deeper Pathways of the
Web by Miki Shima and Charles Chase
ISBN 1-891845-15-2
ISBN 978-1-891845-15-4

CHINESE MEDICAL OBSTETRICS by Bob Flaws
ISBN 1-891845-30-6
ISBN 978-1-891845-30-7

CHINESE MEDICAL PALMISTRY: Your Health in
Your Hand by Zong Xiao-fan & Gary Liscum
ISBN 0-936185-64-3
ISBN 978-0-936185-64-4

CHINESE MEDICAL PSYCHIATRY: A Textbook and
Clinical Manual by Bob Flaws and James Lake, MD
ISBN 1-845891-17-9
ISBN 978-1-845891-17-8

CHINESE MEDICINAL TEAS: Simple, Proven, Folk
Formulas for Common Diseases & Promoting Health
by Zong Xiao-fan & Gary Liscum
ISBN 0-936185-76-7
ISBN 978-0-936185-76-7

CHINESE MEDICINAL WINES & ELIXIRS
by Bob Flaws Revised Edition
ISBN 0-936185-58-9
ISBN 978-0-936185-58-3

CHINESE PEDIATRIC MASSAGE THERAPY: A
Parent's & Practitioner's Guide to the Prevention &
Treatment of Childhood Illness by Fan Ya-li
ISBN 0-936185-54-6
ISBN 978-0-936185-54-5

CHINESE SCALP ACUPUNCTURE
by Jason Jishun Hao & Linda Lingzhi Hao
ISBN 1-891845-60-8
ISBN 978-1-891845-60-4

CHINESE SELF-MASSAGE THERAPY: The Easy Way
to Health by Fan Ya-li
ISBN 0-936185-74-0
ISBN 978-0-936185-74-3

THE CLASSIC OF DIFFICULTIES: A Translation of the
Nan Jing translation by Bob Flaws
ISBN 1-891845-07-1
ISBN 978-1-891845-07-9

A CLINICIAN'S GUIDE TO USING GRANULE
EXTRACTS by Eric Brand
ISBN 1-891845-51-9
ISBN 978-1-891845-51-2

A COMPENDIUM OF CHINESE MEDICAL
MENSTRUAL DISEASES by Bob Flaws
ISBN 1-891845-31-4
ISBN 978-1-891845-31-4

CONCISE CHINESE MATERIA MEDICA
by Eric Brand and Nigel Wiseman
ISBN 0-912111-82-8
ISBN 978-0-912111-82-7

CONTEMPORARY GYNECOLOGY: An Integrated Chinese-Western Approach by Lifang Liang
ISBN 1-891845-50-0
ISBN 978-1-891845-50-5

CONTROLLING DIABETES NATURALLY WITH CHINESE MEDICINE by Lynn Kuchinski
ISBN 0-936185-06-3
ISBN 978-0-936185-06-2

CURING ARTHRITIS NATURALLY WITH CHINESE MEDICINE by Douglas Frank & Bob Flaws
ISBN 0-936185-87-2
ISBN 978-0-936185-87-3

CURING DEPRESSION NATURALLY WITH CHINESE MEDICINE by Rosa Schnyer & Bob Flaws
ISBN 0-936185-94-5
ISBN 978-0-936185-94-1

CURING FIBROMYALGIA NATURALLY WITH CHINESE MEDICINE by Bob Flaws
ISBN 1-891845-09-8
ISBN 978-1-891845-09-3

CURING HAY FEVER NATURALLY WITH CHINESE MEDICINE by Bob Flaws
ISBN 0-936185-91-0
ISBN 978-0-936185-91-0

CURING HEADACHES NATURALLY WITH CHINESE MEDICINE by Bob Flaws
ISBN 0-936185-95-3
ISBN 978-0-936185-95-8

CURING IBS NATURALLY WITH CHINESE MEDICINE by Jane Bean Oberski
ISBN 1-891845-11-X
ISBN 978-1-891845-11-6

CURING INSOMNIA NATURALLY WITH CHINESE MEDICINE by Bob Flaws
ISBN 0-936185-86-4
ISBN 978-0-936185-86-6

CURING PMS NATURALLY WITH CHINESE MEDICINE by Bob Flaws
ISBN 0-936185-85-6
ISBN 978-0-936185-85-9

DISEASES OF THE KIDNEY & BLADDER by Hoy Ping Yee Chan, et al.
ISBN 1-891845-37-3
ISBN 978-1-891845-35-6

THE DIVINE FARMER'S MATERIA MEDICA: A Translation of the Shen Nong Ben Cao translation by Yang Shouz-zhong
ISBN 0-936185-96-1
ISBN 978-0-936185-96-5

DUI YAO: THE ART OF COMBINING CHINESE HERBAL MEDICINALS by Philippe Sionneau
ISBN 0-936185-81-3
ISBN 978-0-936185-81-1

ENDOMETRIOSIS, INFERTILITY AND TRADITION-AL CHINESE MEDICINE: A Layperson's Guide by Bob Flaws
ISBN 0-936185-14-7
ISBN 978-0-936185-14-9

THE ESSENCE OF LIU FENG-WU'S GYNECOLOGY by Liu Feng-wu, translated by Yang Shou-zhong
ISBN 0-936185-88-0
ISBN 978-0-936185-88-0

EXTRA TREATISES BASED ON INVESTIGATION & INQUIRY: A Translation of Zhu Dan-xi's Ge Zhi Yu Lun translation by Yang Shou-zhong
ISBN 0-936185-53-8
ISBN 978-0-936185-53-8

FIRE IN THE VALLEY: TCM Diagnosis & Treatment of Vaginal Diseases by Bob Flaws
ISBN 0-936185-25-2
ISBN 978-0-936185-25-5

FULFILLING THE ESSENCE: A Handbook of Traditional & Contemporary Treatments for Female Infertility by Bob Flaws
ISBN 0-936185-48-1
ISBN 978-0-936185-48-4

FU QING-ZHU'S GYNECOLOGY trans. by Yang Shou-zhong and Liu Da-wei
ISBN 0-936185-35-X
ISBN 978-0-936185-35-4

GOLDEN NEEDLE WANG LE-TING: A 20th Century Master's Approach to Acupuncture by Yu Hui-chan and Han Fu-ru, trans. by Shuai Xue-zhong
ISBN 0-936185-78-3
ISBN 978-0-936185-78-1

A HANDBOOK OF CHINESE HEMATOLOGY by Simon Becker
ISBN 1-891845-16-0
ISBN 978-1-891845-16-1

A HANDBOOK OF TCM PATTERNS & THEIR TREATMENTS   Second Edition by Bob Flaws & Daniel Finney
ISBN 0-936185-70-8
ISBN 978-0-936185-70-5

A HANDBOOK OF TRADITIONAL CHINESE DERMATOLOGY by Liang Jian-hui, trans. by Zhang Ting-liang & Bob Flaws
ISBN 0-936185-46-5
ISBN 978-0-936185-46-0

A HANDBOOK OF TRADITIONAL CHINESE GYNE-COLOGY by Zhejiang College of TCM, trans. by Zhang Ting-liang & Bob Flaws
ISBN 0-936185-06-6 (4th edit.)
ISBN 978-0-936185-06-4

A HANDBOOK of TCM PEDIATRICS by Bob Flaws
ISBN 0-936185-72-4
ISBN 978-0-936185-72-9

THE HEART & ESSENCE OF DAN-XI'S METHODS OF TREATMENT by Xu Dan-xi, trans. by Yang Shou-zhong
ISBN 0-926185-50-3
ISBN 978-0-936185-50-7

HERB TOXICITIES & DRUG INTERACTIONS: A Formula Approach by Fred Jennes with Bob Flaws
ISBN 1-891845-26-8
ISBN 978-1-891845-26-0

IMPERIAL SECRETS OF HEALTH & LONGEVITY by Bob Flaws
ISBN 0-936185-51-1
ISBN 978-0-936185-51-4

INSIGHTS OF A SENIOR ACUPUNCTURIST by Miriam Lee
ISBN 0-936185-33-3
ISBN 978-0-936185-33-0